Workbook
to accompany

Health Careers Today

Third Edition

Judith Gerdin, BSN, MS
Paradise Valley High School
Phoenix, Arizona

 Mosby

An Affiliate of Elsevier

Mosby
An Affiliate of Elsevier
11830 Westline Industrial Drive
St. Louis, MO 63146

Workbook to accompany Health Careers Today, 3rd edition

ISBN-13: 978-0-323-01868-5
ISBN-10:   0-323-01868-8

Vice President, Publishing Director: Sally Schrefer
Editor: Shirley Kuhn
Development Editor: Amy Holmes
Publishing Services Manager: Gayle May

Printed in the United States of America

Last digit is print number: 9   8   7   6   5   4

Preface to the Student

This workbook was designed for use with the textbook *Health Careers Today*. It provides exercises that reinforce the information presented in the textbook and activities that allow you, the student, to demonstrate that material.

The chapters of the workbook are divided into the following sections:

- *Vapid Vocabulary* is a section that provides words from the textbook chapter that may be unfamiliar to you. This section should be completed before the chapter is read to help you understand the content of the chapter.
- *Key Search* and *Key Cryptogram* puzzles allow you to review and use the Key Terms that are found at the beginning of each chapter in the textbook.
- *Abbreviations* presents 10 medical abbreviations that relate to the content of the chapter. This section contains new material for you to learn.
- *Concept Applications* allow you to review and use information from the chapter.
- *Investigations* provide laboratory exercises that apply and expand on the information provided in the textbook. These activities should only be completed under the supervision of a qualified professional.
- The *Critical Thinking Exercises* are included to develop your awareness of health care concerns and expand your thinking skills. These exercises often ask for your opinion and may have more than one correct answer.

Your teacher will give you directions regarding which of these components you are to complete to meet the objectives of your class.

Judith A. Gerdin

Acknowledgments

Throughout the course of my experience in both health care and education, I have been very fortunate to work with highly qualified and dedicated professionals. I am also privileged to have a family that provides me with the support that producing a major work requires.

To both my colleagues and my family, I am grateful. Thank you.

J.G.

Contents

1 Health Care of the Past, Present, and Future

Vapid Vocabulary

Before reading the chapter, challenge your knowledge of words used in the chapter by completing the crossword puzzle of glossary terms.

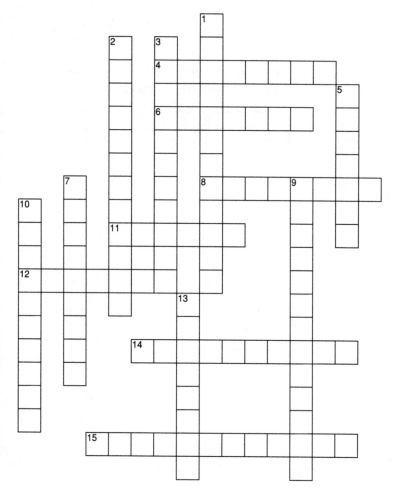

ACROSS

4 Associated with school of higher learning such as a university
6 Person under medical care and treatment
8 Employment or business involving a skill
11 Person who engages the professional services of another
12 Interruption of normal function of the body usually caused by a factor that can be treated such as microorganisms

14 Capable of being transmitted from one person to another
15 Medical doctor specializing in delivery of babies

DOWN
 1 One who has met educational and training requirements to practice health care
 2 Related to factors of both psychologic and social nature
 3 Failure of professional skill or learning that results in injury, loss, or damage
 5 Referring to the central unit of government of the United States
 7 A significant point in development
 9 Pertaining to the society and the effects on it of production, distribution, and consumption of goods and services
10 Document showing that a person is entitled to credit or to exercise official power
13 One who uses goods or services produced by another

Key Cryptogram

Cryptograms are puzzles that include writing in code or cipher. Use the table below to establish the cryptogram key and match the definitions with the correct Key Term from the textbook.

A	B	C	D	E	F	G	H	I	J	K	L	M	N	O	P	Q	R	S	T	U	V	W	X	Y	Z
											4													5	

A.
$\underline{26}\ \underline{22}\ \underline{22}\ \underline{9}\ \underline{6}\ \underline{9}\ \underline{15}\ \underline{L}\quad \underline{1}\ \underline{13}\ \underline{6}\ \underline{26}\ \underline{1}\ \underline{2}\quad \underline{26}\ \underline{22}$

$\underline{9}\ \underline{23}\ \underline{2}\ \underline{9}\ \underline{17}\ \underline{9}\ \underline{23}\ \underline{15}\ \underline{L}\ \underline{21}\quad \underline{14}\ \underline{3}\ \underline{15}\ \underline{L}\ \underline{9}\ \underline{22}\ \underline{9}\ \underline{13}\ \underline{2}$

$\underline{20}\ \underline{26}\quad \underline{24}\ \underline{13}\ \underline{1}\ \underline{22}\ \underline{26}\ \underline{1}\ \underline{12}\quad \underline{6}\ \underline{13}\ \underline{1}\ \underline{20}\ \underline{15}\ \underline{9}\ \underline{23}$

$\underline{21}\ \underline{13}\ \underline{1}\ \underline{17}\ \underline{9}\ \underline{6}\ \underline{13}\ \underline{21}$ means   _____.

B.
$\underline{24}\ \underline{1}\ \underline{13}\ \underline{21}\ \underline{3}\ \underline{20}\ \underline{13}\ \underline{1}\ \underline{12}\ \underline{9}\ \underline{23}\ \underline{13}\ \underline{2}$

$\underline{24}\ \underline{15}\ \underline{Y}\ \underline{12}\ \underline{13}\ \underline{23}\ \underline{20}\quad \underline{21}\ \underline{20}\ \underline{1}\ \underline{3}\ \underline{6}\ \underline{20}\ \underline{3}\ \underline{1}\ \underline{13}\quad \underline{22}\ \underline{26}\ \underline{1}$

$\underline{19}\ \underline{13}\ \underline{15}\ \underline{L}\ \underline{20}\ \underline{19}\quad \underline{6}\ \underline{15}\ \underline{1}\ \underline{13}\quad \underline{21}\ \underline{13}\ \underline{1}\ \underline{17}\ \underline{9}\ \underline{6}\ \underline{13}\ \underline{21}$

$\underline{13}\ \underline{21}\ \underline{20}\ \underline{15}\ \underline{7}\ \underline{L}\ \underline{9}\ \underline{21}\ \underline{19}\ \underline{13}\ \underline{2}\quad \underline{7}\ \underline{Y}\quad \underline{20}\ \underline{19}\ \underline{13}$

‾‾ ‾‾ ‾‾ ‾‾ ‾‾ ‾‾ ‾‾   ‾‾ ‾‾ ‾‾ ‾‾ ‾‾ ‾‾ ‾‾ ‾‾ ‾‾ ‾‾
22 13 21 3 1 15 L   8 26 17 13 1 23 12 13 23 20

means _____

C. ‾‾ ‾‾   ‾‾ ‾‾ ‾‾ ‾‾ ‾‾ ‾‾ ‾‾ ‾‾ ‾‾   ‾‾ ‾‾
   15 23   26 6 6 3 24 15 20 9 26 23   26 1

‾‾ ‾‾ ‾‾ ‾‾ ‾‾ ‾‾ ‾‾ ‾‾ ‾‾ ‾‾   means _____.
24 1 26 22 13 21 21 9 26 23

D. ‾‾ ‾‾ ‾‾ ‾‾ ‾‾ ‾‾ ‾‾   ‾‾ ‾‾ ‾‾   ‾‾ ‾‾ ‾‾ ‾‾ ‾‾ ‾‾
   24 15 Y 12 13 23 20   22 26 1   19 13 15 L 20 19

‾‾ ‾‾ ‾‾ ‾‾   ‾‾ ‾‾ ‾‾ ‾‾ ‾‾ ‾‾ ‾‾ ‾‾, ‾‾ ‾‾ ‾‾ ‾‾ ‾‾
 6 15 1 13   13 18 24 13 23 21 13 21   16 19 9 6 19

‾‾ ‾‾ ‾‾   ‾‾ ‾‾   ‾‾ ‾‾ ‾‾   ‾‾ ‾‾ ‾‾   ‾‾ ‾‾ ‾‾ ‾‾ ‾‾,
12 15 Y   26 1   12 15 Y   23 26 20   26 6 6 3 1

‾‾ ‾‾   ‾‾ ‾‾ ‾‾ ‾‾ ‾‾ ‾‾   ‾‾ ‾‾ ‾‾   ‾‾
 9 23   1 13 20 3 1 23   22 26 1   15

‾‾ ‾‾ ‾‾ ‾‾ ‾‾ ‾‾ ‾‾ ‾‾ ‾‾   ‾‾ ‾‾ ‾‾ ‾‾ ‾‾ ‾‾ ‾‾   ‾‾ ‾‾
21 24 13 6 9 22 9 13 2   24 15 Y 12 13 23 20   9 23

‾‾ ‾‾ ‾‾ ‾‾ ‾‾ ‾‾ ‾‾   means _____.
15 2 17 15 23 6 13

E. ‾‾ ‾‾ ‾‾ ‾‾ ‾‾   ‾‾ ‾‾ ‾‾ ‾‾ ‾‾ ‾‾ ‾‾ ‾‾ ‾‾   ‾‾ ‾‾
   L 13 8 15 L   15 3 20 19 26 1 9 20 Y   20 26

‾‾ ‾‾ ‾‾ ‾‾ ‾‾ ‾‾ ‾‾   ‾‾ ‾‾   ‾‾ ‾‾ ‾‾ ‾‾ ‾‾ ‾‾ ‾‾ ‾‾   means
24 13 1 22 26 1 12   15 23   15 6 20 9 17 9 20 Y

_____.

F. ‾‾ ‾‾ ‾‾ ‾‾ ‾‾ ‾‾ ‾‾ ‾‾
   26 22 22 9 6 9 15 L

‾‾ ‾‾ ‾‾ ‾‾ ‾‾ ‾‾ ‾‾ ‾‾ ‾‾ ‾‾ ‾‾ ‾‾ ‾‾   ‾‾ ‾‾
15 3 20 19 26 1 9 25 15 20 9 26 23   26 1

‾‾ ‾‾ ‾‾ ‾‾ ‾‾ ‾‾ ‾‾ ‾‾   means _____.
15 24 24 1 26 17 15 L

G. $\frac{}{2}\ \frac{}{26}\ \frac{}{6}\ \frac{}{3}\ \frac{}{12}\ \frac{}{13}\ \frac{}{23}\ \frac{}{20}\ \frac{}{15}\ \frac{}{20}\ \frac{}{9}\ \frac{}{26}\ \frac{}{23}\quad \frac{}{26}\ \frac{}{22}$

$\frac{}{19}\ \frac{}{15}\ \frac{}{17}\ \frac{}{9}\ \frac{}{23}\ \frac{}{8}\quad \frac{}{12}\ \frac{}{13}\ \frac{}{20}\quad \frac{}{6}\ \frac{}{13}\ \frac{}{1}\ \frac{}{20}\ \frac{}{15}\ \frac{}{9}\ \frac{}{23}$

$\frac{}{21}\ \frac{}{20}\ \frac{}{15}\ \frac{}{23}\ \frac{}{21}\ \frac{}{5}\ \frac{}{1}\ \frac{}{2}\ \frac{}{21}$ means _____.

H. $\frac{}{26}\ \frac{}{6}\ \frac{}{6}\ \frac{}{3}\ \frac{}{24}\ \frac{}{15}\ \frac{}{20}\ \frac{}{9}\ \frac{}{26}\ \frac{}{23}\quad \frac{}{20}\ \frac{}{19}\ \frac{}{15}\ \frac{}{20}$

$\frac{}{1}\ \frac{}{13}\ \frac{}{14}\ \frac{}{3}\ \frac{}{9}\ \frac{}{1}\ \frac{}{13}\ \frac{}{21}\quad \frac{}{21}\ \frac{}{24}\ \frac{}{13}\ \frac{}{6}\ \frac{}{9}\ \frac{}{15}\ \frac{}{L}\ \frac{}{9}\ \frac{}{25}\ \frac{}{13}\ \frac{}{2}$

$\frac{}{10}\ \frac{}{23}\ \frac{}{26}\ \frac{}{16}\ \frac{}{L}\ \frac{}{13}\ \frac{}{2}\ \frac{}{8}\ \frac{}{13}\quad \frac{}{15}\ \frac{}{23}\ \frac{}{2}\quad \frac{}{26}\ \frac{}{22}\ \frac{}{20}\ \frac{}{13}\ \frac{}{23}$

$\frac{}{L}\ \frac{}{26}\ \frac{}{23}\ \frac{}{8}\quad \frac{}{15}\ \frac{}{23}\ \frac{}{2}\quad \frac{}{9}\ \frac{}{23}\ \frac{}{20}\ \frac{}{13}\ \frac{}{23}\ \frac{}{21}\ \frac{}{9}\ \frac{}{17}\ \frac{}{13}$

$\frac{}{15}\ \frac{}{6}\ \frac{}{15}\ \frac{}{2}\ \frac{}{13}\ \frac{}{12}\ \frac{}{9}\ \frac{}{6}\quad \frac{}{20}\ \frac{}{1}\ \frac{}{15}\ \frac{}{9}\ \frac{}{23}\ \frac{}{9}\ \frac{}{23}\ \frac{}{8}$ means

_____.

I. $\frac{}{L}\ \frac{}{13}\ \frac{}{8}\ \frac{}{15}\ \frac{}{L}\quad \frac{}{2}\ \frac{}{9}\ \frac{}{21}\ \frac{}{24}\ \frac{}{3}\ \frac{}{20}\ \frac{}{13},\quad \frac{}{L}\ \frac{}{15}\ \frac{}{16}\ \frac{}{21}\ \frac{}{3}\ \frac{}{9}\ \frac{}{20}$

means _____.

J. $\frac{}{17}\ \frac{}{26}\ \frac{}{6}\ \frac{}{15}\ \frac{}{20}\ \frac{}{9}\ \frac{}{26}\ \frac{}{23},\quad \frac{}{15}\ \frac{}{6}\ \frac{}{20}\ \frac{}{9}\ \frac{}{17}\ \frac{}{9}\ \frac{}{20}\ \frac{}{Y}\quad \frac{}{9}\ \frac{}{23}$

$\frac{}{16}\ \frac{}{19}\ \frac{}{9}\ \frac{}{6}\ \frac{}{19}\quad \frac{}{26}\ \frac{}{23}\ \frac{}{13}\quad \frac{}{24}\ \frac{}{15}\ \frac{}{1}\ \frac{}{20}\ \frac{}{9}\ \frac{}{6}\ \frac{}{9}\ \frac{}{24}\ \frac{}{15}\ \frac{}{20}\ \frac{}{13}\ \frac{}{21}$

means _____.

Abbreviations

Use the appendix at the back of the textbook to define the following abbreviations.

1. AIDS _____

2. AMA _____

3. CEO _____

4. DRG _____

5. FDA _____

6. HMO _____

7. MD _____

8. PhD _____

9. PPO _____

10. TB _____

Just the Facts

1. Some medications in current use come from herbs and plants that were used in the past including _ _ _ _ _ _ _ and _ _ _ _ _ _ _ _ _ _.

2. The focus of health care has shifted from prevention of contagious diseases to those that are
   related to lifestyle choices such as _ _ _ _ _ _, _ _ _ _ _
   _ _ _ _ _ _, and _ _ _ _ _ disease.

3. The agency of the federal government that oversees the nation's health care is the
   _ _ _ _ _ _ _ _ _ _ _ _ _ _ _ _ _ _ _ _ _.

4. Some of the influences on health care in the United States include the _ _ _ _ _ _ _,
   supply and _ _ _ _ _ _, and _ _ _ _ _ _ _ _ _ _.

5. Some of the opportunities that are provided to health care workers include new _ _
   _ _ _ _ _ _ _ _, a stable _ _ _ _ _ _ _ and employment, and the ability
   to move to new locations.

6. The credentials that may be required for employment in the health care industry include
   _ _ _ _ _ _ _ _ _, _ _ _ _ _ _ _ _ _ _ _ _ _ _, and
   _ _ _ _ _ _ _ _ _ _ _ _ _.

7. One of the influences that will affect health care in the future is the growing population of
   _ _ _ _ _ _ _.

8. Innovations that will affect health care of the future include _ Ⓞ _ _ _ _ _ _ _ _ _ _ _ _ _ and telemedicine.

9. The Internet provides information about Ⓞ _ _ _ _ _ _ Ⓞ _ _ _ _ _ _ _ _ that may not be from a reputable practitioner.

10. Health care workers of the future must be _ Ⓞ _ _ _ _ _ _, able to solve _ Ⓞ _ _ _ _ _ _, and willing to continue to _ Ⓞ _ _ _.

Use the circled letters to form the answer to this jumble. Clue: What is one characteristic of the United States that separates it from all other industrial nations?

_ _   _ _ _ _ _ _ _ _ _ _   _ _ _ _ _ _ _   _ _ _ _

Concept Applications

Historical Perspectives

Choose 25 of the milestones of health care progress from Box 1-1, Medical Milestones, in the text-book to construct a timeline of health care progress in Figure 1-1.

Trends of Today

Using the local newspaper, determine which health career positions are available in your area. Use your observations to answer the following questions.

1. Which job category has the most advertisements for unfilled job opportunities?

_____

_____

_____

2. Use the textbook to write a description of the job duties of the position you identified in question 1.

_____

_____

_____

3. Why do you think there is such a high demand for the career you identified in question 1?

_____

_____

_____

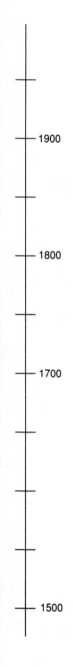

Figure 1-1

Careers of the Future

According to studies by the U.S. Department of Labor, the fastest-growing occupations or those projected to have the largest numerical increases in employment between 2000 and 2010 include those listed below.

Use the textbook and the internet to describe the job duties of four of the occupations listed below.

Education or Training	Profession or Occupation
First professional degree	Chiropractor Optometrist Pharmacist Physician Surgeon Veterinarian
Doctoral degree	Biological scientist Medical scientist
Master's degree	Audiologist Mental health and substance abuse social worker Physical therapist Psychologist Speech-language pathologist
Work experience and bachelor's degree (or higher)	Medical and health services manager
Associate degree	Dental hygienist Medical records and health information technician Occupational therapist assistant Physical therapist assistant Registered nurse Veterinary technologist and technician
Post-secondary vocational training	Licensed practical and licensed vocational nurse Respiratory therapy technician Surgical technologist
On-the-job training (1 to 12 months)	Ambulance driver Dental assistant Medical assistant Pharmacy technician Social and human services assistant
On-the-job training (0 to 1 month)	Home health aide Personal and home care aide Physical therapist aide Veterinary assistant and laboratory animal care-taker

1. Career: _____

  _____

  _____

  _____

2. Career: _____

_____

_____

_____

3. Career: _____

_____

_____

_____

4. Career: _____

_____

_____

_____

Critical Thinking

Reducing the Threat of Disease

Based on projections by the Public Health Service, Americans could reduce the more than $250 billion cost of health care by 70% by making lifestyle changes and using preventive care. The top five leading conditions that result in death in the United States are heart disease, cancer, stroke, chronic lung disease, and accidents. They can all be influenced significantly by nutrition, exercise, and the use of safety precautions.

List one lifestyle change that would reduce the risk of developing each of the five top killers. Suggest one excuse that a person might use when choosing not to make the change.

1. Heart disease

_____

_____

Excuse for not changing:

_____

_____

_____

2. Cancer

_____

_____

Excuse for not changing:

_____

_____

_____

3. Stroke

_____

_____

Excuse for not changing:

_____

_____

4. Chronic lung disease

_____

_____

Excuse for not changing:

_____

_____

5. Accident

_____

_____

Excuse for not changing:

_____

_____

_____

The Cost of Testing

In today's health care industry, physicians use more those 1500 tests to help diagnose health conditions. The tests conducted in the United States cost $150 billion each year. That amount is approximately one third of the $450 billion spent on health care yearly. The American Medical Association estimates that 15% of all medical costs result from what is called "defensive medicine," or testing designed to prevent malpractice suits.

Some suggestions that have been proposed to reduce unnecessary expenditures include:
- Limiting the liability of the medical doctor in the case of misdiagnosis
- Establishing guidelines for signs and symptoms that require further testing
- Providing insurance reimbursement only for tests commonly used given specific signs and symptoms

Answer the following questions regarding methods to reduce health care costs.

1. Propose at least one more method that might be used to reduce the number of unnecessary tests performed.

   _____

   _____

   _____

2. Examine each proposal and explain why you believe it would or would not reduce the number of unnecessary tests.

   a. Limiting medical liability

   _____

   _____

   b. Establishing guidelines for necessary tests

   _____

   _____

   c. Limiting reimbursement for tests

   _____

   _____

3. Discuss the possibility of cost containment in one other area of health care.

   _____

   _____

   _____

2 Interpersonal Dynamics and Communication

Vapid Vocabulary

Before reading the chapter, challenge your knowledge of words used in the chapter by completing the crossword puzzle of glossary terms.

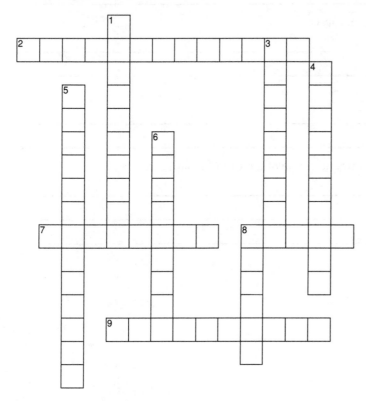

ACROSS

2 Resulting from improvements in productivity of machines
7 The return of information about the result of a process or activity; an evaluative response
8 Reward or punishment due
9 State or quality of being adequately or well qualified; ability

DOWN

1 Not to be cleared up; answer is not found
3 Bold and definite in character
4 Sympathy for another's distress and a desire to remove it
5 Involving relations between people
6 Positiveness of opinion; unwarranted or arrogant
8 Environment; setting

Key Cryptogram

Cryptograms are puzzles that include writing in code or cipher. Use the table below to establish the cryptogram key and match the definitions with the correct Key Term from the textbook.

A	B	C	D	E	F	G	H	I	J	K	L	M	N	O	P	Q	R	S	T	U	V	W	X	Y	Z
											25													21	

A. __ __ __ __   __ __   __ __ __ __ __ __ __ __ __ __ ,
    19 6 3 26   9 18   24 17 26 18 24 L 16 26 17 17

    __ __ __ __ __ __ __ __ __ __ , __ __ __ __ __ __ __ __ __
    8 4 10 9 19 3 6 16 11 26   9 19   1 26 16 26 19 6 L

    __ __ __ __ __   means _____ .
    14 9 19 3 7

B. __ __ __ __ __ __   __ __ __ __ __ __ __ __   __ __
    4 26 16 3 6 L   10 9 17 8 3 8 9 16   9 19

    __ __ __ __ __ __ __   __ __ __ __   __ __ __ __ __ __   __ __
    18 26 26 L 8 16 1   14 8 3 7   19 26 1 6 19 13   3 9

    __   __ __ __ __   __ __   __ __ __ __ __ __ __ __ __
    6   18 6 11 3   9 19   17 8 3 24 6 3 8 9 16

    means _____ .

C. __ __ __ __ __ __ __ __   __ __
    26 15 11 7 6 16 1 26   9 18

    __ __ __ __ __ __ __ __ __ __ __   means _____ .
    8 16 18 9 19 4 6 3 8 9 16

D. __ __ __ __ __ __   __ __   __ __ __ __ __ __
    1 19 6 13 26 13   9 19   19 6 16 23 26 13

    __ __ __ __ __ __   means _____ .
    17 26 19 8 26 17

E. __ __ __ __ __ __ __ __ __ __ __ __   __ __ __ __ __ __ __
    11 9 4 4 24 16 8 11 6 3 8 16 1   14 8 3 7 9 24 3

    __ __ __ __ __   __ __ __ __ __ __ __ __   means _____ .
    24 17 8 16 1   L 6 16 1 24 6 1 26

F. $\overline{}$ $\overline{}$ $\overline{}$ $\overline{}$ $\overline{}$ $\overline{}$ $\overline{}$ $\overline{}$ $\overline{}$ $\overline{}$ $\overline{}$ $\overline{}$ $\overline{}$ $\overline{}$ $\overline{}$ $\overline{}$ $\overline{}$
   17 26 3 3 L 26 13   3 26 16 13 26 16 11 Y   9 18

$\overline{}$ $\overline{}$ $\overline{}$ $\overline{}$ $\overline{}$ $\overline{}$ $\overline{}$ $\overline{}$ means _____.
   12 26 7 6 20 8 9 19

G. $\overline{}$ $\overline{}$ $\overline{}$ $\overline{}$ $\overline{}$ $\overline{}$ $\overline{}$ $\overline{}$ $\overline{}$ $\overline{}$ $\overline{}$,
   17 26 3   9 18   3 19 6 8 3 17

$\overline{}$ $\overline{}$ $\overline{}$ $\overline{}$ $\overline{}$ $\overline{}$ $\overline{}$ $\overline{}$ $\overline{}$ $\overline{}$ $\overline{}$ $\overline{}$ $\overline{}$ $\overline{}$, $\overline{}$ $\overline{}$ $\overline{}$
   11 7 6 19 6 11 3 26 19 8 17 3 8 11 17   6 16 13

$\overline{}$ $\overline{}$ $\overline{}$ $\overline{}$ $\overline{}$ $\overline{}$ $\overline{}$ $\overline{}$ $\overline{}$ $\overline{}$ $\overline{}$ $\overline{}$ $\overline{}$ $\overline{}$ $\overline{}$ $\overline{}$ $\overline{}$
   12 26 7 6 20 8 9 19 17   3 7 6 3   4 6 23 26

$\overline{}$ $\overline{}$ $\overline{}$ $\overline{}$ $\overline{}$ $\overline{}$ $\overline{}$ $\overline{}$ $\overline{}$ $\overline{}$ $\overline{}$
   9 16 26   10 26 19 17 9 16   6 16

$\overline{}$ $\overline{}$ $\overline{}$ $\overline{}$ $\overline{}$ $\overline{}$ $\overline{}$ $\overline{}$ $\overline{}$ $\overline{}$ means _____.
   8 16 13 8 20 8 13 24 6 L

H. $\overline{}$ $\overline{}$ $\overline{}$ $\overline{}$ $\overline{}$ $\overline{}$ $\overline{}$ $\overline{}$ $\overline{}$ $\overline{}$ $\overline{}$ $\overline{}$ $\overline{}$ $\overline{}$ $\overline{}$ $\overline{}$ $\overline{}$ $\overline{}$
   4 6 16 16 26 19   9 18   11 9 16 13 24 11 3 8 16 1

$\overline{}$ $\overline{}$ $\overline{}$ $\overline{}$ $\overline{}$ $\overline{}$ $\overline{}$ means _____.
   9 16 26 17 26 L 18

I. $\overline{}$ $\overline{}$ $\overline{}$ $\overline{}$ $\overline{}$ $\overline{}$ $\overline{}$ $\overline{}$ $\overline{}$ $\overline{}$ $\overline{}$ $\overline{}$
   19 26 L 6 3 8 16 1   3 9   9 19

$\overline{}$ $\overline{}$ $\overline{}$ $\overline{}$ $\overline{}$ $\overline{}$ $\overline{}$ $\overline{}$ $\overline{}$ $\overline{}$ $\overline{}$ $\overline{}$ $\overline{}$ $\overline{}$ $\overline{}$ $\overline{}$ $\overline{}$
   11 9 16 17 8 17 3 8 16 1   9 18   14 9 19 13 17

$\overline{}$ $\overline{}$ $\overline{}$ $\overline{}$ $\overline{}$ $\overline{}$ $\overline{}$ $\overline{}$ means _____.
   9 19   17 9 24 16 13 17

J. $\overline{}$ $\overline{}$ $\overline{}$ $\overline{}$ $\overline{}$ $\overline{}$ $\overline{}$ $\overline{}$ $\overline{}$ $\overline{}$ $\overline{}$ $\overline{}$ $\overline{}$ $\overline{}$ $\overline{}$ $\overline{}$ $\overline{}$ $\overline{}$ $\overline{}$ $\overline{}$
   13 8 17 3 8 16 11 3 8 20 26   5 24 6 L 8 3 8 26 17

$\overline{}$ $\overline{}$ $\overline{}$ $\overline{}$ $\overline{}$ $\overline{}$ $\overline{}$ $\overline{}$ $\overline{}$ $\overline{}$ $\overline{}$ $\overline{}$
   3 7 6 3   4 6 23 26   24 10   6 16

$\overline{}$ $\overline{}$ $\overline{}$ $\overline{}$ $\overline{}$ $\overline{}$ $\overline{}$ $\overline{}$ $\overline{}$ $\overline{}$ means _____.
   8 16 13 8 20 8 13 24 6 L

Abbreviations

Use the appendix at the back of the textbook to define the following abbreviations.

1. cc _____

2. CHO _____

3. chol _____

4. GI _____

5. MRI _____

6. nsg _____

7. pm _____

8. pt _____

9. q.d. _____

10. WHO _____

Just the Facts

1. Health care workers must be able to communicate _ _ _ _ _ _ _ _ _ _ _ _ _ _ _,
   provide _ _ _ _ _ _ _ _ _ _ _ _ _, and use _ _ _ _ _ _ _ _ _ _
   _ _ _ _ _ equipment.

2. Some helpful tips in interpersonal relationships include communicating _ _ _ _,
   acting _ _ _ _ _ _ _ _ _ _ _ _ _ _ _ _, and demonstrating
   _ _ _ _ _ _ _ _ _ _ _.

3. How a person thinks determines his or her _ _ _ _ _ _ _ _ _ and
   _ _ _ _ _ _ _ _ _ _ _ that result from an event.

4. Character is the sum of the _ _ _ _ _ _ _ _ _, attitudes, and
   _ _ _ _ _ _ _ that a person shows to others.

5. The World Health Organization defines health as a state of _ _ _ _ _ _ _ _ _,
   _ _ _ _ _ _ _, and social well-being.

6. Many diseases cause symptoms of general stress including fatigue, weight loss, aches, and
   _ _ _ _ _ _ _ _ _ _ _ _ _ _ _ _ _ problems.

7. Stress may be managed with proper _ _ _ _ _ _ _ _ _ _ _, _ _ _ _ _
   _ _ _ _ _, _ _ _ _ _ _ _ _ _ _ techniques, and changes in personal
   behavior.

8. Critical thinking includes intentional application of _ _ ◯ _ _ ◯ _ _, higher order thinking skills.

9. Assertive communication allows each person to express feelings, opinions, and beliefs in a _ _ _ _ _ ◯ _ _ _ _ and _ _ _ _ ◯ _ _ _ _ _ ◯ manner.

10. With effective communication, the _ ◯ _ _ _ _ and ◯ _ _ _ _ _ _ _ _ messages are the same.

Use the circled letters to form the answer to this jumble. Clue: On what foundation is a person's value system formed?

_ _

Concept Applications

Personal Grooming Checklist

Good grooming habits are essential in all areas of health care. Take this short survey to evaluate your personal grooming habits. Identify three areas of personal grooming that you would like to improve. Chart your effort to improve over the next 4 weeks in the spaces provided.

Yes	No	Grooming or Health Habit
		I maintain my health by getting at least 6 hours of sleep each night.
		I maintain my health by eating a well-balanced diet.
		I maintain my health by having good posture.
		I maintain my health by seeing a doctor when necessary.
		I maintain my health by having my eyes checked when necessary.
		I bathe every day.
		I shampoo my hair regularly.
		I keep my hair styled in a neat manner (away from my face and off my collar).
		I use deodorant every day.
		I maintain my skin by using lotion and treating skin disorders as needed.
		I shave daily (men) or as needed (women) to remove unsightly hair.
		I wear clean undergarments daily.
		I wear all appropriate undergarments.
		I brush my teeth regularly (at least twice daily).
		I floss my teeth regularly (at least once daily).
		I use mouthwash regularly (at least once daily).
		I visit the dentist at least once yearly.
		I keep my fingernails clean and trimmed evenly.
		I wear clothes that fit properly.
		I wear clothes that are clean and pressed.
		I keep my clothes mended.
		I change my socks or stockings daily to reduce foot odor.
		I wear shoes that are clean and fit properly.

continued

Yes	No	Grooming or Health Habit
		I wear a clean uniform each day, which includes my nametag, watch, black pen, and writing paper.
		I wear shoes with my uniform that are nonskid, sturdy, and have low heels.
		I wear minimal jewelry with my uniform.
		I wear no perfume or cologne with my uniform to avoid irritating clients who are ill.

List the three ways you can improve your personal health or grooming.

1. _____
_____
_____

2. _____
_____
_____

3. _____
_____
_____

Date	Goal Progress Report
Current date	Goal:
1-Week evaluation	
2-Week evaluation	
3-Week evaluation	
4-Week evaluation	

Date	Goal Progress Report
Current date	Goal:
1-Week evaluation	
2-Week evaluation	
3-Week evaluation	
4-Week evaluation	

Date	Goal Progress Report
Current date	Goal:
1-Week evaluation	
2-Week evaluation	
3-Week evaluation	
4-Week evaluation	

Problem-Solving Models

Use these sample stories to complete the problem-solving model in the space provided.

Problem 1: You receive your first test back in chemistry class. The grade is a D. You had taken notes during the class lectures, skimmed the chapter, and looked over your notes the night before the test. You had done most of the homework assignments and earned a C grade on them. You know that a grade of D in chemistry could prevent you from going on to an advanced program or college. You want to improve your grade.

Step 1: Recognize that a problem exists. What is the problem?	
Step 2: Clarify the issue. List who is involved and where, when, and how the problem occurred. What other factors affect it?	
Step 3: Identify alternative methods for resolving the problem.	
Step 4: Choose the best method for resolving the problem and implement it. (You may use your imagination to finish the problem.)	
Step 5: Evaluate the results of the method chosen. (You may use your imagination to finish the problem.)	

Problem 2: Describe a problem that you face in your school, work, or home situations. Use the problem-solving method to develop a solution.

Step 1: Recognize that a problem exists. What is the problem?	
Step 2: Clarify the issue. List who is involved and where, when, and how the problem occurred. What other factors affect it?	
Step 3: Identify alternative methods for resolving the problem.	
Step 4: Choose the best method for resolving the problem and implement it.	
Step 5: Evaluate the results of the method chosen	

Investigations

Observing Communication Behaviors

Review Box 2-5 in the textbook. Use the guidelines describing attitudes and behaviors that are barriers to effective communication to observe conversations in your daily life. Describe at least five examples of barriers you observed in your own communication or that of others.

1. _____

_____

2. _____

_____

3. _____

_____

4. _____

_____

5. _____

_____

Questions

1. Which of the barriers that you observed can be easily changed?

_____

_____

_____

2. Why do you think that people use barriers in their communication with others?

_____

_____

_____

Practicing Telephone Etiquette

Work with a partner for this activity. Play the role of the client with your partner acting as the receptionist in the following situations. The "client" may add information to the situation if desired. The "receptionist" may ask for any additional information needed. Evaluate your telephone technique by having the "receptionist" repeat the information gathered after all of the situations have been completed.

Situation 1: Your daughter, aged 2 years, has been running a fever of 102° all night. The child has been crying, and you have had very little sleep. You want to make an appointment to see the doctor as soon as possible.

Situation 2: You are calling to try to find a new veterinarian for your dog. A friend gave you the name of this practitioner. You would like to know the price of the services, the number of veterinarians and hours that service is available, and how long they have been practicing. It is also important to you that emergency care is available. If the information you receive is satisfactory, you will make an appointment to vaccinate your dog.

Situation 3: You are calling to make an appointment with the dentist for an annual check-up. You have been experiencing some cold sensations by one of your right molars, which you think may be a problem. It is important that you do not miss school for the appointment.

Situation 4: You are working as an assistant on a hospital unit. Although answering the phone is not part of your job, you are the only one in the area when the phone rings. The caller is a doctor wanting to leave admission orders for a client.

Situation 5: Invent and convey a message to your partner.

Questions

1. Was any part of the meaning of your message lost in your communication?

_____

_____

_____

2. How can you improve your ability to communicate clearly?

_____

_____

_____

Critical Thinking

Time Management

Use the chart below to record the time you usually spend on the following activities of daily living each day. Convert these estimated times to weekly percentages and complete Figure 2-1. Each week has 10,080 minutes.

Activity	Time in Minutes
Sleeping	
Eating	
Dressing/undressing	
Exercising	
Reading/study	
School/work	
Leisure activity	
Shopping/errands	
Other:	
Other:	

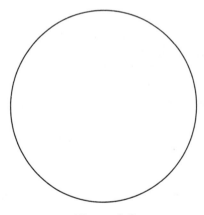

Figure 2-1

Questions

1. On which activity do you spend the most time?

   _____

   _____

   _____

2. On which activity do you spend more time than you would prefer?

_____

_____

_____

3. On which activity do you spend less time than you would prefer?

_____

_____

_____

4. Are there any changes that you might make in your daily activities that would allow you to spend more time on the activities you prefer?

_____

_____

_____

3 *Safety Practices*

Vapid Vocabulary

Before reading the chapter, challenge your knowledge of words used in the chapter by completing the crossword puzzle of glossary terms.

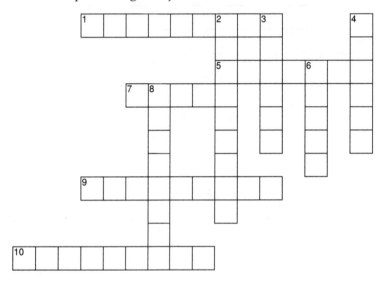

ACROSS

  1 Method used to discover cause and nature of an illness
  5 Capable of destroying or burning
  7 Solid or liquid in gaseous state such as steam
  9 Form assumed by some bacteria that is resistant to heat, drying, and chemicals
 10 Arrangement of a group of points or objects along a line

DOWN

  2 Process by which glands produce and add chemical substances into the blood; substance, such as saliva, mucus, tears, bile, or a hormone, that is secreted
  3 Matter ejected from the respiratory tract through the mouth
  4 Carrier that transfers an infective agent from one host to another
  6 Poisonous
  8 Present in the air; may be carried in respiratory droplets

Key Cryptogram

Cryptograms are puzzles that include writing in code or cipher. Use the table below to establish the cryptogram key and match the definitions with the correct Key Term from the textbook.

A	B	C	D	E	F	G	H	I	J	K	L	M	N	O	P	Q	R	S	T	U	V	W	X	Y	Z
											10													13	

A. ‾‾ ‾‾ ‾‾ ‾‾ ‾‾ ‾‾ ‾‾ ‾‾ ‾‾   ‾‾ ‾‾ ‾‾ ‾‾   ‾‾ ‾‾ ‾‾ ‾‾ ‾‾
11 15 5 11 18 4 24 22 14   18 1 4 18   7 2 L L 11

‾‾ ‾‾ ‾‾ ‾‾ ‾‾ ‾‾ ‾‾ ‾‾ ‾‾ ‾‾ ‾‾ ‾‾ ‾‾   ‾‾ ‾‾ ‾‾ ‾‾ ‾‾ ‾‾
25 2 22 8 26 26 8 12 4 24 2 11 25 11   14 20 22 14 9 18

‾‾ ‾‾ ‾‾ ‾‾ ‾‾ ‾‾ ‾‾   ‾‾ ‾‾ ‾‾   ‾‾ ‾‾ ‾‾ ‾‾ ‾‾ ‾‾   means _____.
16 2 8 15 11 14 11   4 24 3   11 9 26 8 14 11

B. ‾‾ ‾‾ ‾‾ ‾‾ ‾‾ ‾‾ ‾‾ - ‾‾ ‾‾ ‾‾ ‾‾ ‾‾ ‾‾ ‾‾
3 2 11 14 4 11 14 22 4 15 11 2 24 12

‾‾ ‾‾ ‾‾ ‾‾ ‾‾ ‾‾ ‾‾ ‾‾ ‾‾ ‾‾ ‾‾ ‾‾   means _____.
25 2 22 8 26 26 8 12 4 24 2 11 25

C. ‾‾ ‾‾ ‾‾ ‾‾ ‾‾ ‾‾ ‾‾   ‾‾ ‾‾ ‾‾ ‾‾   ‾‾ ‾‾ ‾‾ ‾‾ ‾‾ ‾‾ ‾‾ ‾‾ ‾‾ ;
23 8 14 14 3 26 25   23 8 26 25   2 24 23 14 22 18 2 26 24

‾‾ ‾‾ ‾‾   ‾‾ ‾‾ ‾‾ ‾‾ ‾‾ ‾‾ ‾‾   ‾‾ ‾‾ ‾‾ ‾‾   ‾‾ ‾‾
18 1 14   25 14 18 1 26 3 11   15 11 14 3   18 26

‾‾ ‾‾ ‾‾ ‾‾ ‾‾ ‾‾ ‾‾   ‾‾ ‾‾ ‾‾   ‾‾ ‾‾ ‾‾ ‾‾ ‾‾ ‾‾   ‾‾ ‾‾
9 8 14 16 14 24 18   18 1 14   11 9 8 14 4 3   26 23

‾‾ ‾‾ ‾‾ ‾‾ ‾‾ ‾‾ ‾‾ ‾‾ ‾‾ ‾‾ ‾‾ ‾‾ ‾‾   means _____.
25 2 22 8 26 26 8 12 4 24 2 11 25 11

D. ‾‾ ‾‾   ‾‾ ‾‾ ‾‾ ‾‾ ‾‾ ‾‾ ‾‾ ‾‾ ‾‾ ‾‾   ‾‾ ‾‾ ‾‾ ‾‾ ‾‾ ‾‾ ‾‾
4 24   2 24 23 14 22 18 2 26 15 11   3 2 11 14 4 11 14

‾‾ ‾‾   ‾‾ ‾‾ ‾‾ ‾‾ - ‾‾ ‾‾ ‾‾ ‾‾ ‾‾ ‾‾
26 23   19 4 8 25   5 L 26 26 3 14 3

‾‾ ‾‾ ‾‾ ‾‾ ‾‾ ‾‾ ‾‾   means _____.
4 24 2 25 4 L 11

E. ‾‾ ‾‾ ‾‾   ‾‾ ‾‾ ‾‾ ‾‾ ‾‾ ‾‾ ‾‾ ‾‾ ‾‾ ‾‾   ‾‾ ‾‾ ‾‾
22 3 22   12 15 2 3 14 L 2 24 14 11   23 26 8

$\overline{2}\ \overline{24}\ \overline{23}\ \overline{14}\ \overline{22}\ \overline{18}\ \overline{2}\ \overline{26}\ \overline{24}\quad \overline{22}\ \overline{26}\ \overline{24}\ \overline{18}\ \overline{8}\ \overline{26}\ \overline{L}$

$\overline{4}\ \overline{9}\ \overline{9}\ \overline{L}\ \overline{2}\ \overline{14}\ \overline{3}\quad \overline{18}\ \overline{26}\quad \overline{9}\ \overline{4}\ \overline{18}\ \overline{2}\ \overline{14}\ \overline{24}\ \overline{18}\ \overline{11}$

$\overline{19}\ \overline{2}\ \overline{18}\ \overline{1}\quad \overline{7}\ \overline{24}\ \overline{26}\ \overline{19}\ \overline{24}\quad \overline{26}\ \overline{8}$

$\overline{11}\ \overline{15}\ \overline{11}\ \overline{9}\ \overline{14}\ \overline{22}\ \overline{18}\ \overline{14}\ \overline{3}\quad \overline{2}\ \overline{24}\ \overline{23}\ \overline{14}\ \overline{22}\ \overline{18}\ \overline{2}\ \overline{26}\ \overline{24}\ \overline{11}$

means _____.

F. $\overline{11}\ \overline{26}\ \overline{2}\ \overline{L},\quad \overline{25}\ \overline{4}\ \overline{7}\ \overline{14}\quad \overline{15}\ \overline{24}\ \overline{22}\ \overline{L}\ \overline{14}\ \overline{4}\ \overline{24},\quad \overline{26}\ \overline{8}$

$\overline{2}\ \overline{24}\ \overline{23}\ \overline{14}\ \overline{22}\ \overline{18}\quad \overline{19}\ \overline{2}\ \overline{18}\ \overline{1}\quad \overline{9}\ \overline{4}\ \overline{18}\ \overline{1}\ \overline{26}\ \overline{12}\ \overline{14}\ \overline{24}\ \overline{11}$

means _____.

G. $\overline{22}\ \overline{3}\ \overline{22}\quad \overline{12}\ \overline{15}\ \overline{2}\ \overline{3}\ \overline{14}\ \overline{L}\ \overline{2}\ \overline{24}\ \overline{14}\ \overline{11}\quad \overline{23}\ \overline{26}\ \overline{8}$

$\overline{2}\ \overline{24}\ \overline{23}\ \overline{14}\ \overline{22}\ \overline{18}\ \overline{2}\ \overline{26}\ \overline{24}\quad \overline{22}\ \overline{26}\ \overline{24}\ \overline{18}\ \overline{8}\ \overline{26}\ \overline{L}$

$\overline{18}\ \overline{1}\ \overline{4}\ \overline{18}\quad \overline{4}\ \overline{8}\ \overline{14}\quad \overline{4}\ \overline{9}\ \overline{9}\ \overline{L}\ \overline{2}\ \overline{14}\ \overline{3}\quad \overline{18}\ \overline{26}$

$\overline{4}\ \overline{L}\ \overline{L}\quad \overline{5}\ \overline{26}\ \overline{3}\ \overline{Y}\quad \overline{23}\ \overline{L}\ \overline{15}\ \overline{2}\ \overline{3}\ \overline{11}\quad \overline{26}\ \overline{23}\quad \overline{4}\ \overline{L}\ \overline{L}$

$\overline{9}\ \overline{4}\ \overline{18}\ \overline{2}\ \overline{14}\ \overline{24}\ \overline{18}\ \overline{11}\quad \overline{4}\ \overline{L}\ \overline{L}\quad \overline{26}\ \overline{23}\quad \overline{18}\ \overline{1}\ \overline{14}$

$\overline{18}\ \overline{2}\ \overline{25}\ \overline{14}$ means _____.

H. $\overline{11}\ \overline{15}\ \overline{5}\ \overline{11}\ \overline{18}\ \overline{4}\ \overline{24}\ \overline{22}\ \overline{14}\quad \overline{18}\ \overline{1}\ \overline{4}\ \overline{18}\quad \overline{3}\ \overline{14}\ \overline{18}\ \overline{14}\ \overline{8}\ \overline{11}$

$\overline{18}\ \overline{1}\ \overline{14}\quad \overline{12}\ \overline{8}\ \overline{26}\ \overline{19}\ \overline{18}\ \overline{1}\quad \overline{26}\ \overline{23}$

$\overline{25}\ \overline{2}\ \overline{22}\ \overline{8}\ \overline{26}\ \overline{26}\ \overline{8}\ \overline{12}\ \overline{4}\ \overline{24}\ \overline{2}\ \overline{11}\ \overline{25}\ \overline{11}$ means _____.

I.

$\overline{23}\ \overline{8}\ \overline{14}\ \overline{14}\quad\overline{23}\ \overline{8}\ \overline{26}\ \overline{25}\quad\overline{L}\ \overline{2}\ \overline{16}\ \overline{2}\ \overline{24}\ \overline{12}$

$\overline{25}\ \overline{2}\ \overline{22}\ \overline{8}\ \overline{26}\ \overline{26}\ \overline{8}\ \overline{12}\ \overline{4}\ \overline{24}\ \overline{2}\ \overline{11}\ \overline{25}\ \overline{11}$ means _____.

J.

$\overline{15}\ \overline{24}\ \overline{2}\ \overline{18}\quad\overline{18}\ \overline{1}\ \overline{4}\ \overline{18}\quad\overline{15}\ \overline{11}\ \overline{14}\ \overline{11}\quad\overline{11}\ \overline{18}\ \overline{14}\ \overline{4}\ \overline{25}$

$\overline{15}\ \overline{24}\ \overline{3}\ \overline{14}\ \overline{8}\quad\overline{9}\ \overline{8}\ \overline{14}\ \overline{11}\ \overline{11}\ \overline{15}\ \overline{8}\ \overline{14}\quad\overline{18}\ \overline{26}$

$\overline{11}\ \overline{18}\ \overline{14}\ \overline{8}\ \overline{2}\ \overline{L}\ \overline{2}\ \overline{21}\ \overline{14}\quad\overline{25}\ \overline{4}\ \overline{18}\ \overline{14}\ \overline{8}\ \overline{2}\ \overline{4}\ \overline{L}\ \overline{11}$

means _____.

Abbreviations

Use the appendix at the back of the textbook to define the following abbreviations.

1. ADL _____
2. BSI _____
3. CDC _____
4. dx _____
5. HICPAC _____
6. NIOSH _____
7. OBRA _____
8. OSHA _____
9. pt _____
10. UP _____

Just the Facts

1. The three elements that must be present for infection to occur include
   _ _ _ _ _ _ _ _ _ _ _ _ _ _ _ _, a susceptible host, and a means of
   _ _ _ _ _ _ _ _ _ _ _ _.

2. Infection may be _ _ _ _ _ _ _ _ _ _ _ _ _ or
   _ _ _ _ _ _ _ _ _ _ _ _ _, local or general.

3. _ Ⓞ _ _ _ _ _ _ precautions are applied to all patients at all times and include all body fluids except perspiration.

4. The primary method of protection against infection is good
_ _ Ⓞ _ _ _ _ _ _ _ _ _ technique.

5. The most common method of transfer of pathogens causing serious illness in health care workers is contact with a _ _ Ⓞ _ _ _ _ _ _ _ _ _ _ _ _ _ _ Ⓞ _ _ or _ _ _ _ _ instrument.

6. _ _ _ _ _ Ⓞ _ is the absence of disease-causing microorganisms.

7. OSHA establishes and enforces standards of Ⓞ _ _ _ _ _ for the workplace.

8. Ⓞ _ _ _ Ⓞ _ _ _ _ _ _ _ _ refers to the way the body is moved to prevent injury to oneself and to others.

9. The three elements that must be present for a fire to occur are Ⓞ _ _ _ _ _ _, _ _ Ⓞ _, and _ _ Ⓞ _.

10. Infectious and hazardous waste may be disposed of in the Ⓞ _ _ _ _ _ system or by Ⓞ _ _ _ _ _ _ _ _ _ _ _ _.

Use the circled letters to form the answer to this jumble. Clue: What are the isolation precautions based on specific types of illness called?

_ _ _ _ _ _ _ _ _ _ _ _ _ _ _-_ _ _ _ _ _

Investigations

Handwashing

Read all directions before beginning this activity. Laboratory activities should be performed only under the supervision of a qualified professional.

Equipment and Supplies

Paper towels
Sink
Scrub brush (optional)
Soap
Ultraviolet light indicator
Ultraviolet light

Directions

1. Cover your hands with a spray or lotion that is only visible under ultraviolet light. Allow solution to dry.
2. Following the skill list procedure found in the textbook, wash and dry your hands with water.
3. Observe your hands briefly under the ultraviolet light to determine if any indicator was missed. Record your results.
4. Perform the activity again using soap and water to compare the effectiveness of this technique in removing the indicator.
5. Observe your hands briefly under the ultraviolet light to determine if any indicator was missed. Record your results.
6. Perform the activity again using water, soap, and a surgical scrub brush to compare the effectiveness of this technique in removing the indicator.
7. Observe your hands briefly under the ultraviolet light to determine if any indicator was missed. Record your results.
8. Continue washing your hands, if necessary, until all of the indicator has been removed.
9. Replace all equipment and supplies in the designated area.

Materials Used	Observations
Water only	
Soap and water	
Soap, water, and brush	

Questions

1. Did you wash all areas of your hands equally well? If not, what areas did you miss?

   _____
   _____
   _____

2. How did the effectiveness of washing with water alone to washing with soap and water compare?

   _____
   _____
   _____

3. How did the effectiveness of washing with soap and water to washing with soap, water, and a surgical scrub brush compare?

   _____
   _____
   _____

Critical Thinking

Medical Detecting

This activity is adapted from the VQI (Vector Quest I) series developed by the Iowa Medical Foundation. It allows you to be an epidemiologist, or medical detective. Use the case study to answer the questions.

Case Study: The Attack of the Mutant Vector

The spring of 1990 had been good to Patrick, a child 5 years of age growing up in Des Moines, Iowa. For his birthday in April his father had taken him and five friends to a movie. Patrick received a bike, a pet, plastic turtles, and other presents for his birthday. The next month he started playing organized soccer in a developmental league. After kindergarten classes, Patrick spent his afternoons playing with his friends in a ravine at the end of the dead-end street. If not playing some game in the woods, Patrick could be found teasing his younger sisters.

Around 6:00 A.M. on May 4, Patrick awoke with a terrible pain in his stomach. The pain was so severe he could barely straighten up. As he groaned and made his way to his parents' room he was overcome with both nausea and diarrhea. Patrick had never been so sick in all his life.

What Patrick had was salmonella, or more precisely one of the 1800 strains of the disease first identified by Daniel Salmon. Many of the strains are named after the city where they were first classified such as Salmonella Muenchen or Salmonella Miami.

Tests quickly verified that Patrick was suffering from one of those 1800 variations. What remained a mystery was how he had contracted the disease. Often salmonella is caused by contaminated food yet no other members of his family were ill, and he hadn't eaten anything different than anyone else for more than 2 weeks. This information, for the most part, eliminated a food vector.

But Patrick was not entirely alone; that spring thousands of other people across America were coming down with salmonella. In fact, thousands more cases than usual were reported. It was an epidemic. The Centers for Disease Control and Prevention quickly identified the vector. See if you can solve this case.

Questions:

1. What questions would you like answered to help you determine the source of Patrick's illness?

   _____

   _____

   _____

2. Complete the correlation chart to determine which variables might be involved in Patrick's illness.

Correlation Chart

Variable	Significant	Marginal	Low

3. Hypothesize what you think could have been the vector for Patrick's illness. Do some research if necessary to identify the vector.

_____

_____

_____

4. What technique of personal hygiene could prevent the spread of the bacteria involved in this case study?

_____

_____

_____

4 Legal and Ethical Practices

Vapid Vocabulary

Before reading the chapter, challenge your knowledge of words used in the chapter by completing the crossword puzzle of glossary terms.

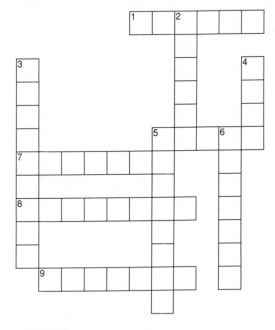

ACROSS

1 Breaking the law, an obligation, or the terms of a contract
5 Range covered by an activity, subject, or topic
7 Permission granted by a person voluntarily and in sound mind
8 About to happen or threatening to happen
9 Unlawful touching of another person without consent

DOWN

2 Belonging to a particular group by descent or culture rather than by nationality
3 An order or official instruction
4 System of accepted laws and regulations that govern procedure of behavior in particular circumstances or within a particular profession
5 Level of quality or excellence that is accepted as the norm or by which actual attainments are judged
6 Using good judgment to consider consequences and to act accordingly

Key Cryptogram

Cryptograms are puzzles that include writing in code or cipher. Use the table below to establish the cryptogram key and match the definitions with the correct Key Term from the textbook.

A	B	C	D	E	F	G	H	I	J	K	L	M	N	O	P	Q	R	S	T	U	V	W	X	Y	Z
											5													8	

A. __ __ __ __ __ __ __ __   __ __   __ __ __ __ __ __ __ __ __ __
   4 12 L 22 15 18 10 19   15 17   13 4 18 10 1 18 13 L 12 6

__ __   __ __ __ __ __   __ __ __   __ __ __ __ __   means _____
17 2   4 18 19 26 15   22 10 3   16 4 17 10 19

B. __ __ __ __ __ __ __ __   __ __ __ __ __ __ __ __ __ __ __ __ __
  24 12 4 7 22 L L Y   1 17 25 25 20 10 18 1 22 15 18 10 19

__ __ __ __ __ __ __ __ __   __ __ __ __ __ __ __ __ __ __
6 17 25 12 15 26 18 10 19   20 10 15 4 20 15 26 2 20 L

__ __ __   __ __ __ __ __ __ __   __ __ __ __ __
22 10 3   26 22 4 25 2 20 L   22 7 17 20 15

__ __ __ __ __ __ __   __ __ __ __ __ __ __   means _____
22 10 17 15 26 12 4   13 12 4 6 17 10

C. __ __ __ __ __ __ __   __ __ __ __   __ __ __ __   __ __
  3 12 22 L 18 10 19   16 18 15 26   16 26 22 15   18 6

__ __ __ __   __ __   __ __ __,
19 17 17 3   17 4   7 22 3

__ __ __ __ __ __ __ __ __ __ __   __ __ __ __ __   __ __ __ __
3 12 15 12 4 25 18 10 18 10 19   25 17 4 22 L   3 20 15 Y

__ __ __   __ __ __ __ __ __ __ __ __ __   means _____
22 10 3   17 7 L 18 19 22 15 18 17 10

D. __ __ __ __ __ __ __   __ __ __ __ __ __ __ __ __ __ __   means
  L 12 19 22 L L Y   4 12 6 13 17 10 6 18 7 L 12

_____

E. __ __ __ __ __ __ __   __ __   __ __ __ __ __ __   means _____
  13 4 18 24 22 15 12   17 4   6 12 1 4 12 15

F. __ __ __ __ __ __ __ __ __ __ __ __ __
  1 17 25 25 20 10 18 1 22 15 18 10 19

6 17 25 12 15 26 18 10 19   20 10 15 4 20 15 26 2 20 L

22 10 3   26 22 4 25 2 20 L   22 7 17 20 15

22 10 17 15 26 12 4   13 12 4 6 17 10   18 10

16 4 18 15 18 10 19   means _____

G. 2 22 18 L 20 4 12   17 2

13 4 17 2 12 6 6 18 17 10 22 L   6 11 18 L L   17 4

L 12 22 4 10 18 10 19   15 26 22 15   4 12 6 20 L 15 6

18 10   18 10 9 20 4 Y,   L 17 6 6,   17 4

3 22 25 22 19 12   means _____

H. 2 22 18 L 20 4 12   15 17   12 21 12 1 20 15 12   15 26 12

1 22 4 12   15 26 22 15   22   4 12 22 6 17 10 22 7 L 12

13 12 4 6 17 10   12 21 12 4 1 18 6 12 6   means _____

I. 3 12 4 18 24 18 10 19   22 20 15 26 17 4 18 15 Y   2 4 17 25

17 4   2 17 20 10 3 12 3   17 10   L 22 16   means _____

J. 6 1 18 12 10 1 12   17 4   13 26 18 L 17 6 17 13 26 Y

17 2   L 22 16   means _____

Abbreviations

Use the appendix at the back of the textbook to define the following abbreviations.

1. AHA _____

2. AMA _____

3. ANA _____

4. APA _____

5. CAHEA _____

6. CEO _____

7. DHSS _____

8. DNR _____

9. HIPAA _____

10. JCAHO _____

Just the Facts

1. Ethical practices include respect for ◯_ _ _ _ _ _ _ _, _ _ ◯_ _ _ _ and _ _ _ ◯_ _ differences of the clients and other workers.

2. Morals are based on the experience, religion, and philosophy of the
   _ ◯_ _ ◯_ _ _ _ _ _ and _ _ _ _ _ _ _ ◯.

3. Workers in every health occupation are legally ◯_ _ _ _ _ _ _ _ _ _ _ (liable) for their behavior and the care given.

4. The duties that may be performed by the health care worker depend on the level of
   ◯_ _ _ _ _ _ _ _ and _ _ _ _ ◯_ _ _ _ of the worker.

5. It is _ _ ◯_ _ _ _ _ _ _ _ _ to perform skills for which the health care worker does not have education and training.

6. In 1996, a federal law was passed to protect individually identifiable health information using
   _ _ _ _ _ _ _ _ _ _ _ technology.

7. The Privacy of Individually _ _ _ _ _ _ ◯_ _ _ _ _ Health Information standards protect _ _ _ ◯_ _ _ records and ◯_ _ _ _ _ _ _ _
   _ _ ◯_ _ _ information.

8. Two types of advance directives are the _ ◯_ _ _ _ _ ◯_ _ and
   _ _ _ ◯_ of _ _ _ ◯_ _ _ ◯.

9. _ _ _ _ O _ _ _ in health care must be precise, clear, and concise.

10. The client's health information is communicated using _ _ _ _ _ _ O _ _ and
    _ _ _ _ _ O _ _ _.

Use the circled letters to form the answer to this jumble. Clue: What do the rights of any citizen of the United States include?

_ _ _ _ _ _ _ and _ _ _ _ _ _ _ _ _ _ _ _ _ _ _ _

Concept Applications

In the News

Use a newspaper or magazine article that describes a current legal or ethical case relating to the health care industry. Complete the information regarding the article in the designated spaces.

1. Title of article:

    _____

2. Name of publication:

    _____

3. Date of publication:

    _____

4. What is the legal breach or issue in dispute in the case described in the article?

    _____

    _____

    _____

5. Summarize the plaintiff's point of view in the case.

    _____

    _____

    _____

6. Summarize the defendant's point of view in the case.

    _____

    _____

    _____

7. Predict the outcome of this legal dispute based on the information provided in the article.

    _____

    _____

    _____

Classifying Conduct

In the following situations, identify whether a legal or ethical breach of conduct is described. Circle the word that corresponds to your choice. If the breach is a legal consideration, explain which crime has occurred. Use Box 4-3 in the textbook for reference.

1. A client in the hospital is angry about her care. She rings her bell 10 or more times an hour. You decide that she is just seeking attention and you ignore the bell.

Legal or Ethical

Explanation:

_____

_____

2. You are helping a nurse who is changing a dressing on a client's wound, and you drop the sterile dressing on the floor. You know that no one saw the dressing drop, and you replace it on the sterile tray to save time and avoid getting into trouble.

Legal or Ethical

Explanation:

_____

_____

3. On arriving home, you find that you have accidentally taken a pen and a roll of tape from work. You decide they are not worth returning and place them in your drawer for use at home.

Legal or Ethical

Explanation:

_____

_____

4. You tell your best friend that, in your role as a student health care worker, you saw a student from your school admitted to the hospital due to an overdose. You name the student who was admitted and your friend promises not to tell anyone else about it. Your friend does not tell anyone.

Legal or Ethical

Explanation:

_____

_____

5. You observe a family in the emergency department after an accident in which one of the children was injured. The family acts very dramatically by crying and clinging to the hospital staff. You mimic that family's reaction for your friends during the football game that evening.

Legal or Ethical

Explanation:

_____

_____

Critical Thinking

Planning Legal and Ethical Strategies

Read the following situations that could create legal and ethical dilemmas in the health care setting. Describe how you would handle the situation and justify your answer in the space provided. Discuss your choices with a partner or group as directed by your instructor.

Situation 1: You observe that one of your coworkers routinely takes items such as pens and paper clips home in her pockets. She comments to you that she uses them for her kids and feels that, with her salary, it is the least the facility can contribute to her kids' education.

   1. How would you handle this situation?

_____

_____

   2. What is your reason for your choice of action?

_____

_____

Situation 2: One of the clients, Mrs. Standwell, is often confused and has difficulty with motor functions such as walking. The family has forbidden the institution to restrain her. You find her after she has fallen and bruised her leg.

   1. How would you handle this situation?

_____

_____

   2. What is your reason for your choice of action?

_____

_____

Situation 3: One client in a double room has difficulty hearing and keeps the television volume high. The other roommate complains that the noise gives him a headache.

   1. How would you handle this situation?

_____

_____

   2. What is your reason for your choice of action?

_____

_____

Situation 4: After the morning break, you smell alcohol on the breath of one of your coworkers.

   1. How would you handle this situation?

_____

_____

   2. What is your reason for your choice of action?

_____

_____

Situation 5: One of the clients tells you that no one came into the room or checked on her throughout the night. She states that even her sleeping pill was omitted.

   1. How would you handle this situation?

_____

_____

   2. What is your reason for your choice of action?

_____

_____

Situation 6: Mrs. Cheats asks you to bring her some salt for her breakfast eggs. She does not have a diet card with her tray and no apparent disorder except the use of oxygen by nasal prongs. You bring her the salt. After she has poured salt on the eggs, she laughs and states, "Ha, I'm not supposed to have salt because of my high blood pressure. Boy, are you in trouble."

   1. How would you handle this situation?

_____

_____

   2. What is your reason for your choice of action?

_____

_____

Situation 7: As you are walking by Mrs. Gripe's room you hear one of your coworkers shout, "Shut up and move it or you'll be sorry."

   1. How would you handle this situation?

_____

_____

   2. What is your reason for your choice of action?

_____

_____

Situation 8: One of your clients is confused and frequently wanders out of his room, stating that he is "going home now." You are short of help and have concerns that he will leave the building.

  1. How would you handle this situation?

  _____

  _____

  2. What is your reason for your choice of action?

  _____

  _____

Situation 9: One of your clients is a jeweler and gives you a ring that he made as a token of appreciation for the care you have given to him.

  1. How would you handle this situation?

  _____

  _____

  2. What is your reason for your choice of action?

  _____

  _____

Situation 10: You notice that one of your coworkers seems to get daily care and vital signs done early every day. A little more observation makes you aware that the person is not changing sheets daily and does not really take the vital signs of many of the clients.

  1. How would you handle this situation?

  _____

  _____

  2. What is your reason for your choice of action?

  _____

  _____

You Be the Judge

Verdict 1:

In July 1991, a surgeon at the Osteopathic Medical Center in Fort Worth, Texas, removed the cancerous right lung of Benjamin H. Jones, Jr., aged 59 years. Unfortunately, an altered test report and prodding by a colleague during the operation led to removal of the wrong lung.

After the pathology examination confirmed that a healthy lung had been removed in error, no one informed Mr. Jones as to what had happened. Court records demonstrated that a top official at the hospital was informed of the discrepancy of the cancer screening and surgery results. The official stated that he relied on the doctors to inform Mr. Jones of the mixup.

Two medical experts swore that Mr. Jones would have had a 60% chance of survival even with only the cancerous lung if he had received radiation therapy. At the time of the surgery, the cancer had not spread past the tumor. Mr. Jones died in February 1992.

The Jones family settled out of court for $5.5 million with 7 defendants in a wrongful-death suit. Along with 20 other defendants, the hospital declined to settle.

Mr. Jones began smoking in his teens and quit after suffering a heart attack about 7 years before the surgery.

Questions

1. What was the breach of law in this case?

_____

_____

2. In your opinion, who was legally responsible for Mr. Jones's death and why?

_____

_____

3. What safeguards might be used to prevent this type of mistreatment in a hospital?

_____

_____

4. In your opinion, do you think that the settlement in this case is fair?

_____

_____

Verdict 2:

In September 1993, Fairfax Hospital in Virginia began to appeal a prior federal court's ruling that it must continue to provide life-sustaining treatment for an anencephalic baby born 11 months earlier. The baby was born with a brainstem that supported respiration and heart activity, but had no cortex. Without a cortex, the baby never had consciousness, sensation, or the ability to think.

After birth, the baby was periodically taken from the nursing home in which he lived to the hospital for treatment of respiratory crisis and to be placed on a respirator. The hospital desired to decline care for the baby. The American Academy of Pediatrics also filed a brief supporting the hospital's position that life-sustaining treatment of this baby was inappropriate.

The mother insisted that the baby be kept alive contrary to the recommendations of the doctors and medical ethics board of the hospital. In fact, the abnormality had been detected before birth and the mother had declined abortion. The baby's father, who has never been married to the mother, supported the hospital's position.

The court decided that refusing treatment violated the Americans with Disabilities Act and the mother's 14th amendment right to "bring up children." The cost of the baby's care, approximately $1,500 a day, was provided by the mother's health maintenance organization.

Questions

1. Most cases involving treatment of severely damaged children raise the question of terminating life instead of prolonging life as in this case. What is the central issue in both of these circumstances?

_____

_____

2. Why do you think that the judge gave the most authority in determining care for this baby to the mother?

_____

_____

3. Which of the facts regarding this case do you feel are most important to making a decision about it?

_____

_____

5 *Employability Skills*

Vapid Vocabulary

Before reading the chapter, challenge your knowledge of words used in the chapter by completing the crossword puzzle of glossary terms.

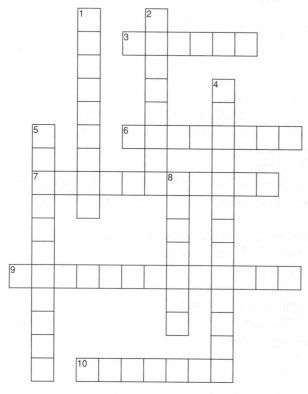

ACROSS

3 Yearly
6 A number more than half the total
7 Expected in the future
9 Giving somebody the freedom to make a decision according to individual circumstances
10 A service such as gas, electricity, or water, provided by a public company

DOWN

1 An accepted standard used in making decisions or judgments about something
2 Cause something, especially an event or process, to begin
4 Pertaining to a representative body
5 Amount of money spent, as a whole or on a particular thing
8 Using as few words as possible to give the necessary information

Key Cryptogram

Cryptograms are puzzles that include writing in code or cipher. Use the table below to establish the cryptogram key and match the definitions with the correct Key Term from the textbook.

A	B	C	D	E	F	G	H	I	J	K	L	M	N	O	P	Q	R	S	T	U	V	W	X	Y	Z
											5													8	

A. __ __ __ __ __   __ __ __ __ __ __ __   __ __
    13 12 7 24 19   5 14 23 23 10 12 Y   16 19

    __ __ __ __ __ __ __ __ __ __ __ __   __ __ __   __ __ __ __
    25 12 16 19 24 5 5 7 16 6 10 L   10 6 22   11 16 12 8

    __ __ __ __ __ __ __ __ __ __   means _____.
    24 9 25 24 12 7 24 6 17 24

B. __ __ __ __ __ __ __ __ __ __ __ __   __ __   __ __ __
    17 16 6 15 12 7 13 14 15 7 16 6   15 16   15 21 24

    __ __ __ __ __ __ __   __ __   __ __ __ __ __ __ __ __ __ __ __ __,
    5 14 25 25 16 12 15   16 19   1 16 3 24 12 6 23 24 6 15

    __ __ __   __ __   __ __ __ __   __ __   __ __
    19 24 24   16 12   22 14 24 5   16 19   10 6

    __ __ __ __ __ __ __ __ __ __ __ __   __ __   __ __ __
    16 12 1 10 6 7 20 10 15 7 16 6   15 16   25 10 Y

    __ __ __   __ __ __ __ __ __ __ __   means _____.
    7 15 5   24 9 25 24 6 5 24 5

C. __ __ __ __ __ __ __   __ __   __ __ __ __ __ __ __ __ __
    5 14 23 23 10 12 Y   16 19   25 12 6 2 24 17 15 24 22

    __ __ __ __ __ __   __ __ __   __ __ __ __ __ __ __ __ __   means _____.
    7 6 17 16 23 24   10 6 22   24 9 25 24 6 5 24 5

D. __ __ __ __ __ __ __   __   __ __ __ __ __ __ __ __ __   means _____.
    22 7 5 17 14 5 5   10   4 14 24 5 15 7 16 6

E. __ __ __ __ __ __ __   __ __ __ __ __ __   means _____.
    16 12 22 24 2 24 22   11 21 16 L 24

F. __ __ __ __ __ __ __ __ __ __ __ __ __ __ __ __ __ __
    10 25 12 16 25 16 5 10 L   19 16 12   10 17 15 7 16 6

means _____.

G. __ __ __ __ __ __ __ __ __ __ __ __ __ __ __ __ __ __ __
    24 6 24 12 1 Y   16 12   10 25 15 7 15 14 22 24   19 16 12

    __ __ __ __ __, __ __ __ __ __ __ __ __ __ __ __   means _____.
    10 17 15 7 16 6   24 6 15 24 12 25 12 7 5 24

H. __ __ __ __ __ __ __ __ __ __ __ __ __ __ __ __ __
    15 16 5 14 5 25 24 6 22   10   5 24 5 5 7 16 6

    __ __ __ __ __ __ __ __ __ __ __ __ __ __ __
    15 16 10 6 16 15 21 24 12   15 7 23 24   16 12

    __ __ __ __ __ __ __ __ __ __ __   means _____.
    25 24 12 23 10 6 24 6 15 L Y

I. __ __ __ __ __ __ __ __ __ __ __ __ __ __ __ __
    L 7 5 15   16 19   15 21 7 6 1 5   15 16   13 24

    __ __ __ __ __ __ __ __ __ __ __ __ __ __ __ __,
    22 16 6 24   16 12   17 16 6 5 7 22 24 12 4 22

    __ __ __ __ __ __ __ __ __ __ __ __ __   means _____.
    25 12 16 1 12 10 23   16 19   11 16 12 8

Abbreviations

Use the appendix at the back of the textbook to define the following abbreviations.

1. AART _____
2. ACSM _____
3. BSN _____
4. CEO _____
5. CMA _____
6. HOSA _____
7. DHSS _____
8. NCHSW _____
9. NIOSH _____
10. VICA _____

Just the Facts

1. In an organization, a group of individuals join together to reach a goal by
   ○ _ _ _ _ _ _ _ _ _ _ _ and division of ○ _ _ _ _ among themselves.

2. Work is a means of self-fulfillment and a method to earn a _ _ ○ _ _ _ and establish
   economic _ _ _ _ _ _ _ _.

3. Benefits of membership in a student organization include the exchange of information
   with others who have similar interests, an opportunity to _ ○ _ _ _ _ _
   _ _ ○ _ _ _ through competition, and a way to develop
   _ _ _ _ _ _ _ _ _ _ ability.

4. One of the elements of an effective group is a clear understanding of its
   ○ _ _ _ _ _ _ _ and _ _ ○ _ _.

5. Parliamentary procedure maintains a sense of order during meetings and ensures that all
   _ _ _ _ _ _ _ have a chance to participate _ _ _ _ _ _ _.

6. Employers use the _ _ _ _ ○ _ _ _ _ _ _ _, résumé, and
   _ _ _ _ _ _ _ _ _ _ to determine who is the best applicant.

7. Many prospective employees do not recognize that the first interview occurs when the
   _ ○ _ _ _ _ _ _ _ _ _ is obtained from the
   _ _ _ _ _ ○ _ _ _ _ _ _.

8. To determine whether an employment opportunity will provide for an employee's needs, a
   _ _ _ _ ○ _ _ _ _ _ _ _ _ _ may be used to determine whether
   these financial goals can be met.

9. Deductions that may be taken from the paycheck before the employee receives it include
   _ _ _ _ _, social security, and _ ○ _ _ _ _ _ _ _ costs.

10. Most people who lose a job after being hired do so because of _ _ _ _ _ _ _ ○
    rather than ○ _ _ _ _ _ _ to do the job.

Use the circled letters to form the answer to this jumble. Clue: What is the first sample of the quality of an employee's work?

_ _ _   _ _ _ _ _ _ _ _ _ _ _ _ _

Concept Applications

Balancing a Checkbook

Use the information provided in Figure 5-1 to balance the checkbook register.

CHECK NO.	DATE	CHECK ISSUED TO OR DEPOSIT RECEIVED FROM	AMOUNT OF CHECK	X	AMOUNT OF DEPOSIT	BALANCE 1058.36
ATM	1/1	Cash-groceries	$100.00	x		$958.36
ATM	1/1	Paycheck		x	$1,523.46	$2,481.82
104	1/5	Telephone	$24.98	x		$2,456.84
105	1/5	Electric	$104.36	x		$2,352.48
106	1/5	Rent	$1,023.00	x		$1,329.48
107	1/10	Car Insurance-6 months	$525.00			$804.48
ATM	1/15	Paycheck			$1,523.46	$2,327.94
108	1/19	Cable-TV	$49.63			$2,278.31
109	1/19	Car payment	$105.68			$2,172.63
ATM	1/19	Cash-groceries	$100.00			$2,072.63

Figure 5-1

Questions

1. Which is the largest expense incurred this month as indicated by the check register?

_____

_____

_____

2. Which of the expenses is a luxury (i.e., not a necessity)?

_____

_____

_____

3. Is the individual with this checkbook living within his or her means? Justify your response using examples from the register.

_____

_____

_____

Creating a Personal Financial Statement

Use Figure 5-2 to create a personal financial statement.

PERSONAL FINANCIAL STATEMENT

Owned:

Cash	$ _____
Securities (stocks, bonds, CDs)	$ _____ *
Real estate	$ _____ *
Automobile	$ _____ *
Furniture	$ _____ *
Receivables (money owed to you)	$ _____
Other	$ _____

Total Owned: $ _____

Owed:

Household bills unpaid	$ _____
Installment payments:	
Automobile	$ _____
Appliances	$ _____
Loans	$ _____
Other	$ _____
Real estate payments	$ _____
Insurance:	
Automobile	$ _____
Personal property	$ _____
Health	$ _____
Other	$ _____
Taxes	$ _____
Other debts	$ _____

Total Owed: $ _____

Total Owned Minus Total Owed Minus Total Worth = $ _____

*Value should be determined by the amount that could be obtained from a quick sale.

Figure 5-2

Questions

1. If your total worth is more than your total debt, what would be a good way to invest the excess?

_____

_____

_____

2. If your total worth is less than your total debt, what would be a source of additional money or an expense that could be cut?

_____

_____

_____

Planning a Budget

Use Figure 5-3 on p. 49 to create a personal budget. Allow at least 5% for savings.

Questions

1. List three expenses that are discretionary, but necessary.

_____

_____

_____

2. Explain why it is more (or less) expensive to eat in a restaurant than at home.

_____

_____

_____

3. What are two ways in which you could reduce your personal expenses without giving up discretionary expenditures that are important to you?

_____

_____

_____

Regular or Fixed Monthly Payments*

Mortgage or rent	$ _____
Automobile payment	$ _____
Automobile insurance	$ _____
Appliance	$ _____
Loan	$ _____
Health insurance	$ _____
Personal property insurance	$ _____
Telephone	$ _____
Utilities (gas or electric)	$ _____
Water	$ _____
Other non-emergency expenses	$ _____

Discretionary or Variable Payments

Clothing, laundry, cleaning	$ _____
Medicine	$ _____
Doctor and dentist	$ _____
Education	$ _____
Dues	$ _____
Gifts and donations	$ _____
Travel	$ _____
Subscriptions	$ _____
Automobile maintenance and gas	$ _____
Spending money and entertainment	$ _____

Food Expenses

Food—at home	$ _____
Food—away from home	$ _____

Taxes

Federal and state income tax	$ _____
Property	$ _____
Other taxes	$ _____

Other

Other	$ _____

TOTAL MONTHLY PAYMENTS $ ____

SAMPLE RECOMMENDED BUDGET EXPENDITURES

Shelter (rent or mortgage)	20%
Food	25%
Clothing	12%
Transportation	12%
Medical and dental	6%
Dues and charities	9%
Education and entertainment	10%
Savings	6%*

----

* Financial advisers recommend that savings should cover expenses for at least 3 months.

Figure 5–3

Planning for Business Meetings

Use Figure 5-4 to complete an agenda for conducting a meeting of your student organization. Conduct a meeting of the organization using the agenda. Use Figure 5-5 to record the secretary's minutes and Figure 5-6 to create a treasurer's report.

AGENDA

BUSINESS ITEM	PERSON RESPONSIBLE
I. Call to Order	Presiding officer: _____
II. Invocation (optional)	Designated officer: _____
III. Pledge of Allegiance (optional)	Presiding officer: _____
IV. Roll Call/Establish Quorum	Secretary: _____
V. Minutes of Previous Meeting	Secretary: _____
VI. Treasurer's Report	Treasurer: _____
VII. Officers' Reports	Vice president: _____
	Others: _____
VIII. Committee Reports A. Standing Committees	Committee chairs: _____
1. Fund Raising	Committee chair: _____
2. Membership	Committee chair: _____
3. Social B. Special	Committee chair: _____
1. Health Fair	Committee chair: _____
2. Field Trip	Committee chair: _____
IX. Unfinished Business	Presiding officer: _____
X. New Business	Presiding officer: _____
XI. Program (optional)	Guest speaker: _____
XII. Announcements	Presiding officer: _____
XIII. Adjournment	Presiding officer: _____

Figure 5-4

Minutes of the Meeting of _____

_____ (date)

The meeting was called to order at _____ (time). The minutes were approved _____ (with/without) changes. The treasurer's report was read and filed for audit.

The _____ (committee or individual) moved to _____

_____ (motion). Discussion was held. The motion (carried/failed to carry) with a majority vote.

The meeting was adjourned at _____ (time).

Respectfully submitted,

_____ (secretary)

Figure 5-5

Treasurer's Report

From _____ (Date) to   (Date) _____

Income
  Membership dues: _____ $ _____
  Fees:_____ $ _____
  Interest:_____ $ _____
  Sales projects: _____ $ _____
  _____ $ _____
  _____ $ _____
  Other: _____ $ _____
  _____ $ _____
  _____ $ _____
  Total income: _____ $ _____
Expenditures:
  Membership dues: _____ $ _____
  Fees:_____ $ _____
  Taxes:_____ $ _____
  Sales projects: _____ $ _____

  _____ $ _____
  _____ $ _____
  Other : _____ $ _____
  _____ $ _____
  _____ $ _____
  Total expenditures:_____ $ _____
  Beginning balance _____ $ _____
  Total income: _____ $ _____
  Sum: _____ $ _____
  Total expenditures: _____ $ _____
  Ending balance: _____ $ _____

Respectfully Submitted,

_____ (Treasurer)

Figure 5-6

Preparing a Résumé

Use Figure 5-7 to complete a draft of a personal data sheet or résumé. Proofread and complete it according to your teacher's instructions.

Personal Data Sheet

Complete the following personal date sheet to assist you in filling out job applications. Employment and educational information should be presented with most current information first. References should be presented in alphabetical order.

_____
(Your Complete Name)

_____
(Address)

_____
(City, State, Zip Code)

_____
(Telephone Number)

Career Objective:
_____

Education
_____
(School, City, State, Years Attended)

_____
(School, City, State, Years Attended)

_____
(School, City, State, Years Attended)

Work Experience
_____
(Place of Employment, Dates Employed)

_____
(Place of Employment, Dates Employed))

Job-Related Skills and Training
_____   _____
_____   _____
_____   _____
_____   _____

Honors and Organizations
_____   _____
_____   _____
_____   _____
_____   _____

Personal Interests and Hobbies
_____   _____
_____   _____
_____   _____
_____   _____

References
_____
(Name, Occupation, Address, City, State, Zip Code, Telephone)

_____
(Name, Occupation, Address, City, State, Zip Code, Telephone)

_____
(Name, Occupation, Address, City, State, Zip Code, Telephone)

Figure 5-7

Completing a Job Application

The job application form provides the employer with the details needed to assess qualifications for employment. It is a personal and professional profile. Use the guidelines provided in the textbook to complete Figure 5-8.

Application for Employment

Date _____

Name _____   Social
                                          Security # _____

Address _____ Zip _____   Telephone
                                                       Number _____

If employed and you are under 18 can you furnish a work permit?   ☐ Yes ☐ No

Are you legally eligible for employment in the U.S.A.?   ☐ Yes ☐ No

Have you worked here before?   ☐ Yes ☐ No   If Yes, when? _____

Are there any hours, shifts or days you cannot or will not work? _____

Are you willing to work overtime if required?   ☐ Yes ☐ No

List friends or relatives working here. _____

Have you ever been convicted of a crime?   ☐ Yes ☐ No (A conviction record will not necessarily be a bar to employment)

EDUCATION

Circle Highest Grade Completed	Grade School 1 2 3 4 5 6 7 8	High School 9 10 11 12	College 1 2 3 4	Graduate 1 2 3 4	Degree Received	Course Of Study
High School	Name and Address					
College(s)						
Graduate/Professional						
Specialized Training, Apprenticeship, Skills						
Honors and Awards and Accreditations						

MILITARY SERVICE RECORD   Have you served in the U.S. Armed Forces? _____ Dates of duty _____

POSITION(S) APPLIED FOR: 1) _____ 2) _____

You must indicate a specific position. Applications stating "ANY POSITION" will not be considered.

Wage or salary requirements $ _____ When can you start? _____

Figure 5–8

WORK HISTORY

If presently employed, may we contact your employer? ( ) Yes ( ) No

(1) **Present or Most Recent Employer**	Address	Phone
Date Started	Starting Salary	Starting Position
Date Left	Salary on Leaving	Position on Leaving
Name and Title of Supervisor		
Description of Duties	Reason for Leaving	

(2) **Previous Employer**	Address	Phone
Date Started	Starting Salary	Starting Position
Date Left	Salary on Leaving	Position on Leaving
Name and Title of Supervisor		
Description of Duties	Reason for Leaving	

(3) **Previous Employer**	Address	Phone
Date Started	Starting Salary	Starting Position
Date Left	Salary on Leaving	Position on Leaving
Name and Title of Supervisor		
Description of Duties	Reason for Leaving	

Figure 5-8 (cont'd)

ADDITIONAL INFORMATION

OTHER QUALIFICATIONS

Summarize special job-related skills and qualifications acquired from employment or other experience.

_____

_____

_____

SPECIALIZED SKILLS   CHECK SKILLS/EQUIPMENT OPERATED

___CRT	___Fax	Other (list):
___PC	___Lotus 1-2-3	_____
___Calculator	___PBX System	_____
___Typewriter	___Wordperfect	_____

State any additional information you feel may be helpful to us in considering your application.

_____

_____

_____

Note to Applicants: DO NOT ANSWER THIS QUESTION UNLESS YOU HAVE BEEN
INFORMED ABOUT THE REQUIREMENTS OF THE JOB FOR WHICH YOU ARE APPLYING.

Are you capable of performing in a reasonable manner, with or without a reasonable accommodation, the activities involved in the job or occupation for which you have applied? A description of the activities involved in such a job or occupation is attached.   ___YES   ___NO

REFERENCES

1. _____   (   ) _____
   (Name)   Phone #

   _____
   (Address)

2. _____   (   ) _____
   (Name)   Phone #

   _____
   (Address)

3. _____   (   ) _____
   (Name)   Phone #

   _____
   (Address)

By my signature below I certify that I have read the above and understand it completely.

_____   _____
Signature   Date

Figure 5-8 (cont'd)

Critical Thinking

Employment Decisions

Employment decisions are made by supervisors to improve the service provided to the clients by an organization. In health care, this means to improve the quality of care given to patients. Use your personal, school, and work experience to explain why each of the following decisions may occur.

Questions

1. The employer keeps an employee on staff that always does a minimal job. Another employee is fired that does a much better job but has a poor attendance record.

    _____

    _____

    _____

2. The employer gives a promotion to an employee with less experience than others. The employee that is promoted has a higher level of education for the job.

    _____

    _____

    _____

3. The employer promotes a person with more experience than others. The employee that is promoted has a lower level of education for the job.

    _____

    _____

    _____

4. The employer tells an employee that his or her work is not being completed in a satisfactory manner. How might the employee handle this situation?

    _____

    _____

    _____

6 Foundation Skills

Vapid Vocabulary

Before reading the chapter, challenge your knowledge of words used in the chapter by completing the crossword puzzle of glossary terms.

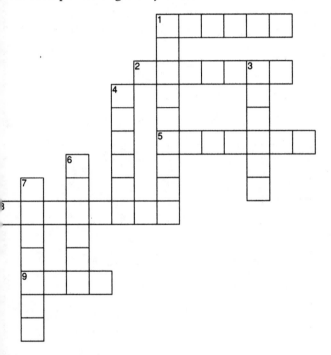

ACROSS

1. Express, communicate
2. Magnify
5. Easy to hear
8. Proportion, amount
9. Pointed end

DOWN

1. Illness, grievance
3. Weak
4. Prescribed amount
6. Acid compound that may be found in urine if fat is used instead of sugar for cell energy
7. Maintain

Key Cryptogram

Cryptograms are puzzles that include writing in code or cipher. Use the table below to establish the cryptogram key and match the definitions with the correct Key Term from the textbook.

A	B	C	D	E	F	G	H	I	J	K	L	M	N	O	P	Q	R	S	T	U	V	W	X	Y	Z
											15													10	

A. ___ ___ ___ ___ ___ ___ ___ ___ ___   ___ ___   ___ ___ ___ ___ ___ ___ ___   ___ ___ ___ ___
11 6 23 8 4 26 9 21 6   2 16   11 18 22 22 26 4 1   12 26 11 8

___ ___ ___   ___ ___ ___ ___ ___ ___ ___ ___ ___ ___   ___ ___   ___ ___ ___ ___ ___ ___ ___ ___
11 8 6   16 26 4 1 6 13 11 26 22 7   11 2   6 20 18 L 21 18 11 6

___ ___ ___ ___,   ___ ___ ___ ___ ___ ___ ___ ___,   ___ ___ ___
7 26 24 6   14 2 13 19 6 13 7   18 4 19

___ ___ ___ ___ ___ ___ ___ ___ ___ ___ ___
23 2 4 7 26 7 11 6 4 23 Y

___ ___   ___ ___ ___ ___ ___ ___ ___ ___   ___ ___ ___ ___ ___ ___ ___ ___ ___ ___ ___   ___ ___
2 16   26 4 11 6 13 4 18 L   7 11 13 21 23 11 21 13 6 7   2 16

___ ___ ___   ___ ___ ___ ___ means _____.
11 8 6   14 2 19 Y

B. ___ ___ ___ ___ ___ ___   ___ ___ ___ ___ ___ ___ ___ ___   ___ ___   ___ ___ ___ ___ ___
7 21 19 19 6 4   7 11 2 22 22 26 4 1   2 16   8 6 18 13 11

___ ___ ___ ___ ___ ___ means _____.
18 23 11 26 2 4

C. ___ ___ ___ ___ ___ ___ ___ ___   ___ ___   ___ ___ ___ ___ ___ ___ ___ ___ ___ ___ ___
22 13 6 7 7 21 13 6   2 16   23 26 13 23 21 L 18 11 26 4 1

___ ___ ___ ___ ___   ___ ___ ___ ___ ___ ___ ___   ___ ___ ___   ___ ___ ___ ___ ___ ___   ___ ___
14 L 2 2 19   18 1 18 26 4 7 11   11 8 6   12 18 L L 7   2 16

___ ___ ___   ___ ___ ___ ___ ___ ___ ___ ___ means _____.
11 8 6   18 13 11 6 13 26 6 7

D. ___ ___ ___ ___ ___   ___ ___ ___ ___ ___ ___ ___   ___ ___ ___ ___ ___ ___
14 L 2 2 19   22 13 6 7 7 21 13 6   19 21 13 26 4 1

___ ___ ___ ___ ___ ___ ___ ___ ___ ___ ___ ___ ___   ___ ___ ___ ___ ___ ___ ___ ___ ___ ___ ___
20 6 4 11 13 26 23 21 L 18 13   23 2 4 11 13 18 23 11 26 2 4

means _____.

E. $\overline{14}$ $\overline{L}$ $\overline{2}$ $\overline{2}$ $\overline{19}$ $\overline{22}$ $\overline{13}$ $\overline{6}$ $\overline{7}$ $\overline{7}$ $\overline{21}$ $\overline{13}$ $\overline{6}$ $\overline{18}$ $\overline{11}$ $\overline{11}$ $\overline{8}$ $\overline{6}$

$\overline{17}$ $\overline{18}$ $\overline{25}$ $\overline{26}$ $\overline{17}$ $\overline{21}$ $\overline{17}$ $\overline{2}$ $\overline{16}$ $\overline{23}$ $\overline{18}$ $\overline{13}$ $\overline{19}$ $\overline{26}$ $\overline{18}$ $\overline{23}$

$\overline{13}$ $\overline{6}$ $\overline{L}$ $\overline{18}$ $\overline{25}$ $\overline{18}$ $\overline{11}$ $\overline{26}$ $\overline{2}$ $\overline{4}$ means _____.

F. $\overline{11}$ $\overline{6}$ $\overline{23}$ $\overline{8}$ $\overline{4}$ $\overline{26}$ $\overline{9}$ $\overline{21}$ $\overline{6}$ $\overline{21}$ $\overline{7}$ $\overline{6}$ $\overline{19}$ $\overline{11}$ $\overline{2}$ $\overline{16}$ $\overline{6}$ $\overline{6}$ $\overline{L}$ $\overline{11}$ $\overline{8}$ $\overline{6}$

$\overline{11}$ $\overline{6}$ $\overline{25}$ $\overline{11}$ $\overline{21}$ $\overline{13}$ $\overline{6}$, $\overline{7}$ $\overline{26}$ $\overline{24}$ $\overline{6}$,

$\overline{23}$ $\overline{2}$ $\overline{4}$ $\overline{7}$ $\overline{26}$ $\overline{7}$ $\overline{11}$ $\overline{6}$ $\overline{4}$ $\overline{23}$ $\overline{Y}$, $\overline{18}$ $\overline{4}$ $\overline{19}$ $\overline{L}$ $\overline{2}$ $\overline{23}$ $\overline{18}$ $\overline{11}$ $\overline{26}$ $\overline{2}$ $\overline{4}$

$\overline{2}$ $\overline{16}$ $\overline{22}$ $\overline{18}$ $\overline{13}$ $\overline{11}$ $\overline{7}$ $\overline{2}$ $\overline{16}$ $\overline{11}$ $\overline{8}$ $\overline{6}$ $\overline{14}$ $\overline{2}$ $\overline{19}$ $\overline{Y}$ $\overline{12}$ $\overline{26}$ $\overline{11}$ $\overline{8}$

$\overline{11}$ $\overline{8}$ $\overline{6}$ $\overline{8}$ $\overline{18}$ $\overline{4}$ $\overline{19}$ $\overline{7}$ means _____.

G. $\overline{22}$ $\overline{6}$ $\overline{13}$ $\overline{11}$ $\overline{18}$ $\overline{26}$ $\overline{4}$ $\overline{26}$ $\overline{4}$ $\overline{1}$ $\overline{11}$ $\overline{2}$ $\overline{11}$ $\overline{8}$ $\overline{6}$ $\overline{18}$ $\overline{22}$ $\overline{6}$ $\overline{25}$ $\overline{2}$ $\overline{13}$

$\overline{22}$ $\overline{2}$ $\overline{26}$ $\overline{4}$ $\overline{11}$ $\overline{6}$ $\overline{19}$ $\overline{6}$ $\overline{4}$ $\overline{19}$ $\overline{2}$ $\overline{16}$ $\overline{11}$ $\overline{8}$ $\overline{6}$ $\overline{8}$ $\overline{6}$ $\overline{18}$ $\overline{13}$ $\overline{11}$

means _____.

H. $\overline{18}$ $\overline{23}$ $\overline{11}$ $\overline{2}$ $\overline{16}$ $\overline{L}$ $\overline{26}$ $\overline{7}$ $\overline{11}$ $\overline{6}$ $\overline{4}$ $\overline{26}$ $\overline{4}$ $\overline{1}$ $\overline{16}$ $\overline{2}$ $\overline{13}$

$\overline{7}$ $\overline{2}$ $\overline{21}$ $\overline{4}$ $\overline{19}$ $\overline{7}$ $\overline{12}$ $\overline{26}$ $\overline{11}$ $\overline{8}$ $\overline{26}$ $\overline{4}$

$\overline{11}$ $\overline{8}$ $\overline{6}$ $\overline{14}$ $\overline{2}$ $\overline{19}$ $\overline{Y}$ means _____.

I. $\overline{4}$ $\overline{6}$ $\overline{23}$ $\overline{6}$ $\overline{7}$ $\overline{7}$ $\overline{18}$ $\overline{13}$ $\overline{Y}$ $\overline{11}$ $\overline{2}$ $\overline{L}$ $\overline{26}$ $\overline{16}$ $\overline{6}$ means _____.

Abbreviations

Use the appendix at the back of the textbook to define the following abbreviations.

1. AP _____

2. ax _____

3. BP _____

4. c/o _____

5. I & O _____

6. P _____

7. pt _____

8. R _____

9. TPR _____

10. VS _____

Just the Facts

1. The basic health assessment may include an interview and _ _ ○ _ _ _ _ _ _ examination to determine functional, ○ _ _ _ _ _ _ _ _, spiritual, and physical _ _ _ _ _ _ _ _ _ _ _ _ _ _ _ _ _ ○.

2. Blood pressure is a measurement of the force of the blood _ _ _ _ _ ○ _ the walls of the _ _ _ _ _ _ _ _ ○ as it circulates through the body.

3. Temperature is the measurement of the balance between the heat _ _ _ _ _ _ _ _ _ and _ _ _ ○ by the body.

4. Pulse is the heartbeat that can be felt (_ _ _ _ _ _ _ _) on surface arteries as the artery walls expand.

5. One respiration includes the _ _ _ _ _ _ _ _ _ _ ○ _ and _ _ _ ○ _ _ _ _ _ _ of a breath.

6. Physical assessment uses techniques of inspection, _ _ _ _ _ ○ _ _ _ _ _ _, palpation, and _ _ _ _ _ _ _ _ ○ _ _.

7. Three systems of measurement used in health care are the _ _ ○ _ _ _ ○ _ _ _, SI (metric), and _ _ _ _ _ _ _ _ _ ○ units.

8. Computers are used in all aspects of health care including laboratory tests and _ _ _ _ ○ _ _ _ _ _ _ _ _ _ _ _ _ _ _ _ ○ _ _ _.

9. The purpose of first aid is to sustain ○ _ _ _ and _ _ _ _ _ _ _ ○ death.

Use the circled letters to form the answer to this jumble. Clue: What are the two measurements made when taking a blood pressure?

_ _ _ _ _ _ _ _ and _ _ _ _ _ _ _ _ _

Concept Applications

Medical Terminology Practice

Use the following prefixes, roots, and suffixes to form 20 medical terms. A transition phrase or vowel may be added to or deleted from the word parts to make the combining form. Define the terms in the space provided.

Naso	Cardio	pnea	ectomy	algia
Psych	Cyst	derm	otomy	centesis
Nephro	Myo	endarter	itis	lysis
Cyan	Brady	lith	ology	ic
Gastro	Oto	orth	oma	gram

Medical Term	Definition
1. _____	_____
2. _____	_____
3. _____	_____
4. _____	_____
5. _____	_____
6. _____	_____
7. _____	_____
8. _____	_____
9. _____	_____
10. _____	_____
11. _____	_____
12. _____	_____
13. _____	_____
14. _____	_____
15. _____	_____
16. _____	_____
17. _____	_____
18. _____	_____
19. _____	_____
20. _____	_____

Graphing Practice

Gather and chart the following data:

A. Height of each student in class in centimeters. Chart as a line graph using the height as the independent variable and the number of students having that height as the dependent variable.

B. Age of each student in months. Chart as a bar graph using the age as the independent variable and the number of students with that age as the dependent variable.

C. Blood pressure and pulse rate of each student in class. Choose a charting method that could be used to compare the blood pressure values in the class with the pulse rates.

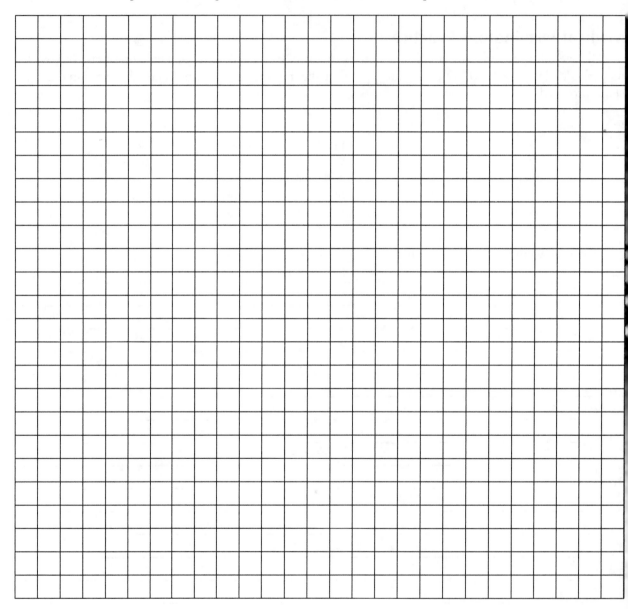

Questions

1. Using the graph, what can you conclude, if anything, about the height of the people in your class?

   _____

   _____

2. Using your graph, what can you conclude, if anything, about the age of the people in your class?

   _____

   _____

3. Using your graph, what can you conclude, if anything, about the relationship of a person's blood pressure and to pulse rate?

   _____

   _____

Investigations

Conducting a Health Assessment

Conduct a health assessment of a fellow student. Chart the appropriate information in Table 6-1.

TABLE 6-1

Student Name	
Height	
Weight	
BP	
Pulse	
Respiration	
Temperature	

Questions

1. Are all of the values you obtained within the normal parameters?

   _____

   _____

2. If any of the values are abnormal, how could these values be improved?

   _____

   _____

Critical Thinking

Review the leading indicators of the healthy person in Box 1-6 of the textbook. Use an Internet search engine and key words to research one of the indicators of health. Use a word processor to produce a paragraph that describes the health indicator. Include the current state of the situation, resources for individual action, and any related information. Print the paragraph from the word-processing program when completed.

One search engine Internet address that can be used is:

http://www.google.com

Key words for one indicator might include:

Tobacco

Health

Incidence

The source of the leading health indicators may be found online at:

http://www.health.gov/healthypeople/LHI/

7 Wellness, Growth, and Development

Vapid Vocabulary

Before reading the chapter, challenge your knowledge of words used in the chapter by completing the crossword puzzle of glossary terms.

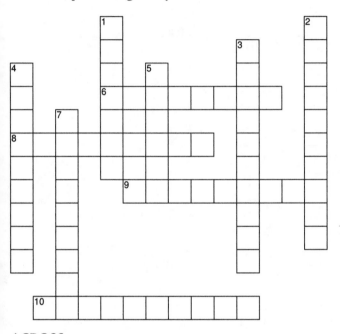

ACROSS

6 Desire to avoid something that is disliked
8 Uninterrupted ordered sequence
9 Complex carbohydrate derived from plant walls
10 Pain-relieving pentapeptide released by brain

DOWN

1 Characterized by a lack of consistency
2 Equal in value
3 Cytoplasm; protein and other materials contained in cells
4 One that comes before; substance used to make another structure
5 Fruit or seed from a leguminous plant; e.g. beans or peas
7 One of the neuropeptides released by the brain that reduces pain

Key Cryptogram

Cryptograms are puzzles that include writing in code or cipher. Use the table below to establish the cryptogram key and match the definitions with the correct Key Term from the textbook.

A	B	C	D	E	F	G	H	I	J	K	L	M	N	O	P	Q	R	S	T	U	V	W	X	Y	Z
										25														16	

A. __ __ __ __ __ __ __ __ __ __ __ __ __ __ __ __ __
   23 5 20 10 1 19 19 20 6 4 11 13 3 2 21 3 24

__ __ __ __ __ __ __ __ __ __ __ __ __ __ __ __ __ __ __ __
24 15 4 5 3 1 24 4 19 11 2 12 15 19 3 24 21 4 2 1 26

__ __ __ __ __ __ Y __ __ __ __ __ __ __ __ __   means _____.
6 20 5 7 20 12 Y 6 15 24 10 4 3 20 24 19

B. __ __ __ __ __ __ __ __ __ __ __ __ L __ __
   24 20 24 20 5 21 11 24 3 10 19 20 L 3 12

__ __ __ __ __ __ __ __ __   means _____.
19 15 7 19 4 11 24 10 1

C. __ __ __ __ __ __ __ __ __ __ __ __ L __ __ __ __ __ __ __ __ __
   21 5 20 15 23 20 6 10 20 26 23 L 1 14 20 5 21 11 24 3 10

__ __ __ __ __ __ __ __ __ __ __ __ __ __ __ __ __ __ __
10 20 26 23 20 15 24 12 19 4 2 11 4 11 5 1 4 2 1

__ __ __ __ __ __ __ __ __ __ __ __ L L
26 11 3 24 23 11 5 4 20 6 10 1 L L

__ __ __ __ __ __ __ __ L __ __ __   means _____.
23 5 20 4 20 23 L 11 19 26

D. __ __ __ __ __ __ __ __, __ __ __ __ __ __ __,
   19 4 11 5 10 2 1 19 19 15 21 11 5 19

__ __ L L __ L __ __ __, __ __ __ __ __ __ __   means _____.
10 1 L L 15 L 20 19 1 11 24 12 21 15 26 19

E. __ __ __ __ __ __ __ __ __ __ __ __ __ __ __ __ __ __ __ __ __ __
   20 5 21 11 24 3 10 10 20 26 23 20 15 24 12 19 24 1 1 12 1 12

__ Y __ __ __ __ __ __ Y __ __ __
7 Y 4 2 1 7 20 12 Y 6 20 5

$\overline{26}\ \overline{1}\ \overline{4}\ \overline{11}\ \overline{7}\ \overline{20}\ \overline{L}\ \overline{3}\ \overline{19}\ \overline{26}$, $\overline{21}\ \overline{5}\ \overline{20}\ \overline{17}\ \overline{4}\ \overline{2}$, $\overline{11}\ \overline{24}\ \overline{12}$

$\overline{12}\ \overline{1}\ \overline{18}\ \overline{1}\ \overline{L}\ \overline{20}\ \overline{23}\ \overline{26}\ \overline{1}\ \overline{24}\ \overline{4}$ means _____.

F. $\overline{23}\ \overline{1}\ \overline{11}\ \overline{5}\ \overline{L}\ \overline{Y}$, $\overline{6}\ \overline{11}\ \overline{4}\ \overline{L}\ \overline{3}\ \overline{13}\ \overline{1}$ $\overline{19}\ \overline{4}\ \overline{1}\ \overline{5}\ \overline{20}\ \overline{3}\ \overline{12}$

$\overline{11}\ \overline{L}\ \overline{10}\ \overline{20}\ \overline{2}\ \overline{20}\ \overline{L}$ $\overline{6}\ \overline{20}\ \overline{15}\ \overline{24}\ \overline{12}$ $\overline{3}\ \overline{24}$ $\overline{11}\ \overline{24}\ \overline{3}\ \overline{26}\ \overline{11}\ \overline{L}$

$\overline{6}\ \overline{11}\ \overline{4}\ \overline{19}$ $\overline{11}\ \overline{24}\ \overline{12}$ $\overline{20}\ \overline{3}\ \overline{L}\ \overline{19}$, $\overline{23}\ \overline{5}\ \overline{1}\ \overline{10}\ \overline{15}\ \overline{5}\ \overline{19}\ \overline{20}\ \overline{5}$

$\overline{20}\ \overline{6}$ $\overline{7}\ \overline{3}\ \overline{L}\ \overline{1}$ $\overline{11}\ \overline{10}\ \overline{3}\ \overline{12}\ \overline{19}$ $\overline{11}\ \overline{24}\ \overline{12}$

$\overline{2}\ \overline{20}\ \overline{5}\ \overline{26}\ \overline{20}\ \overline{24}\ \overline{1}\ \overline{19}$ means _____.

G. $\overline{11}\ \overline{12}\ \overline{3}\ \overline{23}\ \overline{20}\ \overline{19}\ \overline{1}$ $\overline{4}\ \overline{3}\ \overline{19}\ \overline{19}\ \overline{15}\ \overline{1}$; $\overline{5}\ \overline{1}\ \overline{19}\ \overline{1}\ \overline{5}\ \overline{18}\ \overline{1}$

$\overline{19}\ \overline{15}\ \overline{23}\ \overline{23}\ \overline{L}\ \overline{Y}$ $\overline{20}\ \overline{6}$ $\overline{1}\ \overline{24}\ \overline{1}\ \overline{5}\ \overline{21}\ \overline{Y}$ means _____.

H. $\overline{19}\ \overline{15}\ \overline{26}$ $\overline{20}\ \overline{6}$ $\overline{11}\ \overline{L}\ \overline{L}$ $\overline{4}\ \overline{2}\ \overline{1}$ $\overline{23}\ \overline{2}\ \overline{Y}\ \overline{19}\ \overline{3}\ \overline{10}\ \overline{11}\ \overline{L}$

$\overline{11}\ \overline{24}\ \overline{12}$ $\overline{10}\ \overline{2}\ \overline{1}\ \overline{26}\ \overline{3}\ \overline{10}\ \overline{11}\ \overline{L}$ $\overline{23}\ \overline{5}\ \overline{20}\ \overline{10}\ \overline{1}\ \overline{19}\ \overline{19}\ \overline{1}\ \overline{19}$

$\overline{7}\ \overline{Y}$ $\overline{17}\ \overline{2}\ \overline{3}\ \overline{10}\ \overline{2}$ $\overline{11}$ $\overline{L}\ \overline{3}\ \overline{18}\ \overline{3}\ \overline{24}\ \overline{21}$

$\overline{20}\ \overline{5}\ \overline{21}\ \overline{11}\ \overline{24}\ \overline{3}\ \overline{9}\ \overline{1}\ \overline{12}$ $\overline{19}\ \overline{15}\ \overline{7}\ \overline{19}\ \overline{4}\ \overline{11}\ \overline{24}\ \overline{10}\ \overline{1}$ $\overline{3}\ \overline{19}$

$\overline{23}\ \overline{5}\ \overline{20}\ \overline{12}\ \overline{15}\ \overline{10}\ \overline{1}\ \overline{12}$, $\overline{26}\ \overline{11}\ \overline{3}\ \overline{24}\ \overline{4}\ \overline{11}\ \overline{3}\ \overline{24}\ \overline{1}\ \overline{12}$,

$\overline{11}\ \overline{24}\ \overline{12}$ $\overline{4}\ \overline{5}\ \overline{11}\ \overline{24}\ \overline{19}\ \overline{6}\ \overline{20}\ \overline{5}\ \overline{26}\ \overline{1}\ \overline{12}$ $\overline{4}\ \overline{20}$

$\overline{23}\ \overline{5}\ \overline{20}\ \overline{12}\ \overline{15}\ \overline{10}\ \overline{1}$ $\overline{1}\ \overline{24}\ \overline{1}\ \overline{5}\ \overline{21}\ \overline{Y}$ means _____.

I.

$\overline{11}\ \overline{24}\ \overline{Y}$ $\overline{10}\ \overline{20}\ \overline{24}\ \overline{19}\ \overline{4}\ \overline{5}\ \overline{15}\ \overline{10}\ \overline{4}\ \overline{3}\ \overline{18}\ \overline{1}$ $\overline{23}\ \overline{5}\ \overline{20}\ \overline{10}\ \overline{1}\ \overline{19}\ \overline{19}$

$\overline{7}\ \overline{Y}$ $\overline{17}\ \overline{2}\ \overline{3}\ \overline{10}\ \overline{2}$ $\overline{19}\ \overline{3}\ \overline{26}\ \overline{23}\ \overline{L}\ \overline{1}$

$\overline{19}\ \overline{15}\ \overline{7}\ \overline{19}\ \overline{4}\ \overline{11}\ \overline{24}\ \overline{10}\ \overline{1}\ \overline{19}$ $\overline{11}\ \overline{5}\ \overline{1}$ $\overline{10}\ \overline{20}\ \overline{24}\ \overline{18}\ \overline{1}\ \overline{5}\ \overline{4}\ \overline{1}\ \overline{12}$

$\overline{7}\ \overline{Y}$ $\overline{L}\ \overline{3}\ \overline{18}\ \overline{3}\ \overline{24}\ \overline{21}$ $\overline{10}\ \overline{1}\ \overline{L}\ \overline{L}\ \overline{19}$ $\overline{3}\ \overline{24}\ \overline{4}\ \overline{20}$

$\overline{26}\ \overline{20}\ \overline{5}\ \overline{1}$ $\overline{10}\ \overline{20}\ \overline{26}\ \overline{23}\ \overline{L}\ \overline{1}\ \overline{14}$ $\overline{10}\ \overline{20}\ \overline{26}\ \overline{23}\ \overline{20}\ \overline{15}\ \overline{24}\ \overline{12}\ \overline{19}$

means _____.

J.

$\overline{23}\ \overline{5}\ \overline{20}\ \overline{4}\ \overline{1}\ \overline{3}\ \overline{24}\ \overline{19}$, $\overline{10}\ \overline{11}\ \overline{5}\ \overline{7}\ \overline{20}\ \overline{2}\ \overline{Y}\ \overline{12}\ \overline{5}\ \overline{11}\ \overline{4}\ \overline{1}\ \overline{19}$,

$\overline{6}\ \overline{11}\ \overline{4}\ \overline{19}$, $\overline{18}\ \overline{3}\ \overline{4}\ \overline{11}\ \overline{26}\ \overline{3}\ \overline{24}\ \overline{19}$, $\overline{11}\ \overline{24}\ \overline{12}$

$\overline{26}\ \overline{3}\ \overline{24}\ \overline{1}\ \overline{5}\ \overline{11}\ \overline{L}\ \overline{19}$ $\overline{24}\ \overline{1}\ \overline{10}\ \overline{1}\ \overline{19}\ \overline{19}\ \overline{11}\ \overline{5}\ \overline{Y}$ $\overline{6}\ \overline{20}\ \overline{5}$

$\overline{26}\ \overline{11}\ \overline{3}\ \overline{24}\ \overline{4}\ \overline{11}\ \overline{3}\ \overline{24}\ \overline{3}\ \overline{24}\ \overline{21}$ $\overline{20}\ \overline{6}$ $\overline{L}\ \overline{3}\ \overline{6}\ \overline{1}$

means _____.

Abbreviations

Use the appendix at the back of the textbook to define the following abbreviations.

1. Ca^{++} _____

2. cal _____

3. CHO _____

4. chol _____

5. DNR _____

6. Fe^+ _____

7. FF _____

8. H/A _____

9. lb _____

10. wt _____

Just the Facts

1. Wellness may be defined as a state of _ _ _ _ _ O on a continuum from a level of high energy and feeling of well-being to _ _ _ _ O _ _ _ or _ _ O _ _.

2. Fitness may be evaluated by considering muscle strength and endurance, cardiorespiratory _ _ _ _ _ _ O _ _ _, body _ _ _ _ _ _ _ _ _ O _ _, and _ _ _ _ _ _ _ _ _ _ O _ _.

3. Body cells _ O _ _ _ _ _ _ _ _ _ or process food in two ways called anabolism and _ _ _ _ _ O _ _ _ _.

4. The five nutrients that have been identified as being essential to the maintenance of good health are carbohydrates, _ _ _ _ _ _ O _, fats, vitamins, and O _ _ _ _ _ O _ _.

5. _ _ _ _ _ _ _ _ O _ _ _ _ _ are found in all plants that are used as food sources and are the main source of quick or immediate energy used by the body.

6. In addition to meats, _ _ _ _ _ _ _ O _ are found in dried beans, peas, and cheese.

7. _ O _ _ are found in the marbling or white part of meat, cooking oils, salad dressings, and in some milk products such as butter.

8. Stress is the body's _ _ _ _ _ _ _ _ _ _ _ O reaction to demands of everyday life.

9. _ _ _ _ _ O refers to the changes that can be measured in height and weight and in body proportions whereas O _ _ _ _ _ _ _ _ _ _ describes the stages of change in psychologic and social functioning.

10. Five stages of death are _ _ O _ _ _, anger, bargaining, _ _ _ _ _ O _ _ _ _, and acceptance.

Use the circled letters to form the answer to this jumble. Clue: What are two of the common physical disorders linked to stress?

_ _ _ _ _ _ _ _ _ _ _ _ _ _ _ _ _ _ _

Concept Applications

Comparing Nutritional Value

Because of the food labeling legislation, the consumer can compare nutritional value of foods as well as the prices. Use the labels in Figure 7-1 to answer the questions.

Nutrition Facts

Serving Size 1/2 cup (114 g)
Servings Per Container 4

Amount Per Serving
Calories 90   Calories from Fat 30

	% Daily Value*
Total Fat 3 g	5 %
Saturated Fat 0 g	0 %
Cholesterol 0 mg	0 %
Sodium 300 mg	13 %
Total Carbohydrate 13 g	4 %
Dietary Fiber 3 g	12 %
Sugars 3 g	
Protein 3 g	

Vitamin A	80 %	Vitamin C	60 %
Calcium	4 %	Iron	4 %

*Percent daily values are based on a 2000 calorie diet

	Calories	2000	2500
Total Fat	Less than	65 g	80 g
Sat Fat	Less than	20 g	25 g
Cholesterol	Less than	300 mg	300 mg
Sodium	Less than	2400 mg	2400 mg
Total Carbohydrate		300 mg	375 mg
Fiber		25 mg	30 mg

Calories per gram:
Fat 9   Carbohydrate 4   Protein 4

Nutrition Facts

Serving Size 1 bag (56 g)
Servings Per Container 1

Amount Per Serving
Calories 330   Calories from Fat 250

	% Daily Value*
Total Fat 29 g	45 %
Saturated Fat 3 g	14 %
Cholesterol 0 mg	0 %
Sodium 5 mg	0 %
Total Carbohydrate 10 g	3 %
Dietary Fiber 4 g	15 %
Sugars 3 g	
Protein 11 g	

Vitamin A	** %	Vitamin C	** %
Calcium	15 %	Iron	15%

**Less than 2% of Daily Value
*Percent daily values are based on a 2000 calorie die

	Calories	2000	2500
Total Fat	Less than	65 g	80 g
Sat Fat	Less than	20 g	25 g
Cholesterol	Less than	300 mg	300 mg
Sodium	Less than	2400 mg	2400 mg
Total Carbohydrate		300 mg	375 mg
Fiber		25 mg	30 mg

Calories per gram:
Fat 9   Carbohydrate 4   Protein 4

Figure 7-1

Questions

1. Why would one of the food items be better for a person with high blood pressure?

_____

_____

_____

2. Which one of the food items has the best balance of food sources?

_____

_____

_____

3. Which one of the food items would provide a quick source of energy?

_____

_____

_____

4. Explain how the labeling system allows the consumer to compare the food's nutritive value when the serving size is different.

_____

_____

_____

INVESTIGATIONS

Read all directions before beginning this activity. Visit a grocery store to examine labels on food products.

Identify five food products that contain at least 50% by weight of the specified nutrient in each of the categories in Table 7-1. Record the names of the foods in the spaces provided.

Identify five food products that contain at least 50% of the daily value of specified nutrient in each of the categories in Table 7-2. Record the names of the foods in the spaces provided.

Evaluate your list to answer the questions.

TABLE 7-1   Items Containing 50% by Weight

Nutrient	Food Source
Protein	
Carbohydrate	
Fat	

TABLE 7-2   Items Containing 50% Daily Value

Nutrient	Food Source
Total Fat	
Sodium	
Total Carbohydrate	
Protein	
Calcium	
Iron	
Vitamin A	
Vitamin C	
Thiamine	
Niacin	
Folic Acid	

Questions

1. Which items contain the most minerals? To which food group do they belong?

_____

_____

_____

2. Which items contain the most vitamins? To which food group do they belong?

_____

_____

_____

3. How does the nutritive value of the food items chosen compare with the content of carbohydrate, fat and protein?

_____

_____

_____

Assessing Physical Fitness

Physical fitness is the ability to carry out daily tasks easily and to have enough energy to respond to unexpected demands as necessary. Complete each of the four activities to assess your level of physical fitness. Read all the directions before beginning this activity. Laboratory activities should be completed only under the supervision of a qualified professional.

Background Information

Components of Physical Fitness
1. Flexibility—range of movement of joints
2. Strength—greatest amount of work muscles can do in a given period of time
3. Endurance—how well muscles can perform over a time without causing fatigue
4. Cardiovascular endurance—ability of the heart and lungs to deliver oxygen to the body during exercise and then quickly return to a resting rate

DATA CHARTS

Body Flexibility (score in inches)

MEN	WOMEN	RATING
22+	23+	Excellent
17-21	20-23	Good
13-16	17-19	Average
9-12	14-16	Fair
8 or less	13 or less	Poor

Leg Muscle Strength

EXCELLENT - score 5 to 6 inches greater than your height

GOOD - score 2 to 4 inches greater than your height

AVERAGE - score more than 0 to 2 inches greater than your height

FAIR - score equal to your own height

POOR - score less than your own height

MEN	WOMEN	RATING
40+	30+	Excellent
33-39	24-29	Good
29-32	18-24	Average
21-28	11-17	Fair
Less than 21	Less than 11	Poor

Muscle Endurance (number of sit-ups in 1 minute)

PULSE RATE	RATING
70-80	Excellent
81-105	Good
106-119	Average
120-130	Fair
131+	Poor

Pulse Recovery Rate (number of heart beats at the end of 3 minutes of step testing)
Equipment and Supplies
    Mat or blanket
    Step ladder or heavy box
    Stop watch or watch with second hand
    Tape measure or meter stick

Instructions

Activity # 1—Flexibility

1. Do some light stretching exercises to warm up your muscles and prevent injury.
2. Avoid quick, jerking movements. Use gradual, smooth movements.
3. Sit on the floor with your legs straight in front of you. Your heels should be 5 inches apart.
4. Place a yardstick on the floor with the 36-inch mark pointing away from your body. Place the 15-inch mark even with your heels.
5. Slowly reach with both hands as far forward as possible and hold the position.
6. Measure the most distant point that the fingertips reach.
7. Repeat twice more for a total of three trials.

Activity #2—Leg Muscle Strength

1. From the starting point, bend your knees and jump forward (standing broad jump), landing on both feet.
2. Measure your jump in inches.
3. Repeat twice more for a total of three trials.

Activity #3—Muscle Endurance

1. Lie on your back on a mat or blanket with knees slightly bent. Your partner holds your ankles in place.
2. Place your hands behind your head and perform as many sit-ups as you can do in 1 minute.
3. Take care to breathe freely, do not hold your breath. Return to a flat lying position between each sit-up.
4. Repeat twice more for a total of three trials.

Activity #4—Cardiovascular Endurance

1. Take a resting pulse rate for 1 minute and record.
2. While your partner supports the step ladder, step up and down (both feet) continuously for 3 minutes.
3. Step at the rate of 24 steps per minute.
4. Immediately sit down at the end of 3 minutes and take your pulse rate for 1 minute.
5. Rest without talking and monitor your pulse every minute. Record the amount of time needed for your heart to return to its resting rate.

TABLE 7-3   Your Results

Activity #1 - Flexibility	Result
Trial #1	
Trial #2	
Trial #3	
Activity #2 - Muscle Strength	Result
Trial #1	
Trial #2	
Trial #3	
Activity #3 - Muscle Endurance	Result
Trial #1	
Trial #2	
Trial #3	
Activity #4 - Cardiovascular Endurance	Result
Trial #1	
Trial #2	
Trial #3	

Questions

1. Calculate the average result and determine your rating for each of the activities:
   Activity #1 Average _____
   Activity #2 Average _____
   Activity #3 Average _____
   Activity #4 Average _____

2. In which area(s) of physical fitness would you like to improve your performance?

   _____

   _____

   _____

3. What could you do differently in your life to make the improvements listed?

   _____

   _____

   _____

4. What is an aerobic exercise? Give an example of an aerobic exercise.

   _____

   _____

   _____

5. A lifetime sport is one that can be done throughout the lifespan. Describe at least one lifetime sport in which you participate.

   _____

   _____

   _____

6. "Being active naturally" is a phrase used to describe exercise in your daily routine and activities. An example would be to park a distance from the door of the store in order to walk farther to and from the car. Give one example of natural activity in which you participate.

   _____

   _____

   _____

CRITICAL THINKING

Making the Decision to Die

In 1993, Michigan passed a law that makes assisted suicide a felony. This law resulted from the more than 17 assisted suicides involving Dr. Jack Kevorkian. Groups who oppose Dr. Kevorkian's actions question whether all of the suicides were actually voluntary.

When the Oregon Death with Dignity Act was passed in 1994, Oregon became the first state to legalize assisted suicide. However, the law was immediately challenged in the courts. This new legislation allows physicians to assist suicide in cases of terminal illness with a life expectancy of 6 months or less. To obtain lethal medication under the law, the person must be diagnosed as terminal by at least two physicians. Groups that oppose the measure are concerned that people who are ill will choose to commit suicide to prevent expensive medical bills or spare their loved ones from providing care for them.

In 1994 Benito Agrelo, a boy aged 15 years, fought in court for the right to refuse medication. Benny had been born with a malfunctioning liver and had previously undergone two liver transplants. The drugs used to keep Benny's body from rejecting the liver caused migraine headaches and severe leg and back pain. Benny could not read or walk. Benny's physicians felt that Benny could be helped with a third transplant and a change in the dose of the immunosuppressive medication. Using the child-abuse agencies and laws, the physicians forced Benny to return to the hospital. After hearings with a judge, Benny was allowed to return home and refuse treatment. Benny stopped taking the medication in October 1993 and died in August 1994. He reported that these last months were the best months of his life.

Questions

1. In your opinion, is it suicide for a person to refuse treatment such as feeding tubes, or as in the case of Benny, medication?

_____

_____

_____

2. In your opinion, should someone who is terminally ill be allowed to commit suicide?

_____

_____

_____

3. If you had a positive response to question 2, who do you think should be involved in a decision to end someone's life?

_____

_____

_____

4. In your opinion, what criteria determine the value of someone's life?

_____

_____

_____

8 Body Organization

Vapid Vocabulary

Before reading the chapter, challenge your knowledge of words used in the chapter by completing the crossword puzzle of glossary terms.

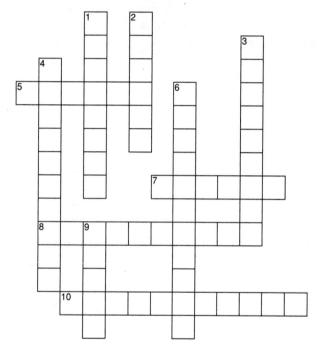

ACROSS

5 Sex of individual, male or female
7 Hollow space
8 Large group of viruses containing RNA
10 Relating to the chemical substances present in living organisms

DOWN

1 One of four regions used to describe location in the abdomen
2 The young of any organism at an early stage of development
3 Set of materials or instrument for a specific operation
4 Pertaining to the extremities or edges; away from the center
6 Wavelengths from 5 to about 400 nanometers of the visible light spectrum
9 Poison produced by animals, plants, or bacteria

Key Search

Find the Key Terms from the chapter in the word search puzzle below. Define each of the terms in the space provided.

```
E  S  I  O  T  I  T  N  T  E  S  C  E  N  M  E  I  U  L  T
T  I  E  T  N  T  A  T  P  I  O  E  U  T  T  D  P  N  E  S
Y  S  E  C  G  G  I  Y  S  N  E  O  I  N  N  H  S  E  S  C
L  A  O  I  G  M  T  T  G  M  E  E  T  N  E  S  D  G  T  I
O  T  I  N  Y  O  T  E  O  O  C  C  O  N  G  Y  S  T  N  R
R  S  Y  S  N  I  N  R  E  P  S  I  O  E  S  A  E  S  I  D
T  O  I  E  T  I  D  L  T  I  M  T  E  D  S  O  S  G  D  U
C  E  G  O  T  N  T  I  E  A  Y  T  N  A  N  I  M  O  D  A
E  M  E  A  Y  S  N  E  I  P  E  S  E  E  M  L  E  D  I  U
L  O  L  S  G  O  T  S  E  A  U  T  O  S  O  M  E  N  A  E
E  H  A  N  A  N  I  I  I  N  Y  S  I  T  V  R  Y  O  N  G
C  O  N  D  I  T  I  O  N  T  E  N  I  O  E  U  E  I  S  E
U  I  N  E  A  T  I  I  I  E  A  Y  N  Y  A  E  O  T  M  E
N  U  O  S  E  A  M  D  C  G  E  U  O  M  E  I  N  A  Y  T
R  T  N  E  I  E  E  S  R  Y  U  T  U  L  H  Y  M  T  G  I
I  T  E  S  N  R  T  O  T  D  I  N  N  I  T  S  I  U  M  E
U  E  M  O  E  I  T  U  M  N  V  A  E  T  N  M  D  M  I  S
E  E  M  H  E  I  T  I  S  I  C  I  Y  O  S  E  I  N  C  N
S  N  E  E  I  Y  I  G  C  R  E  V  I  S  S  E  C  E  R  E
T  E  E  O  O  N  S  I  C  O  S  M  E  T  T  S  S  R  I  S
```

1. Autosome- _____

2. Condition- _____

3. Congenital- _____

4. Disease- _____

5. Dominant- _____

6. Electrolyte- _____

7. Genotype- _____

8. Heredity- _____

9. Homeostasis- _____

10. Mutation- _____

11. Organism- _____

12. Phenotype- _____

13. Recessive- _____

14. Syndrome-_____

Just the Facts

1. The four basic properties of life are reception, _ _ _ _ Ⓞ _ _ _ _ _, reproduction, and _ _ _ Ⓞ _ _ _ _ _ _ _ _ _.

2. The two major types of study of the human body are called _ _ _ Ⓞ _ _ _ _ and _ _ _ _ _ _ Ⓞ _ _ _.

3. _ _ _ _ _ _ _ _ Ⓞ _ _ _ is the tendency of a cell or the whole organism to maintain a state of balance.

4. The four types of tissue in the body are _ _ _ _ _ _ _ _ _ Ⓞ _, _ _ _ _ _ _ _ _ _ Ⓞ _, muscle, and nerve.

5. Ⓞ _ _ _ _ _ _ is the process by which a cell divides to reproduce, creating an identical replica with the same chromosomes.

6. In the process of _ _ Ⓞ _ _ _ _ the cell divides into two parts each with only one half of the chromosomes.

7. _ _ _ _ _ _ _ Ⓞ is the passing on of genetic information that determines the characteristics of an individual person.

8. Abnormal genes or chromosomes cause many disorders, which are therefore called inherited, _ _ _ _ Ⓞ _ _ _ _ _ _, or _ _ _ _ _ _ _ Ⓞ disorders.

9. _ _ Ⓞ _ _ _ is the uncontrolled growth of abnormal cells that tend to spread (metastasize) and invade the tissue around them.

10. Three disorders that have been linked to genetic factors include _ _ _ _ _ _ cancer, _ _ _ _ Ⓞ _ _ _ _ _ _ _ _ _, and _ _ _ _ _ _ _ _ _ Ⓞ _ disease.

Use the circled letters to form the answer to this jumble. Clue: What is the area of the body that contains the stomach, liver, and spleen?

_ _ _ _ _ _ _ _ _ _ _   _ _ _ _ _ _ _

Concept Applications

Identifying Structures of the Cell

Use Figure 8-1 in the textbook to label the diagram of the cell in Figure 8-1. In the spaces provided in Table 8-1, describe the function of each part.

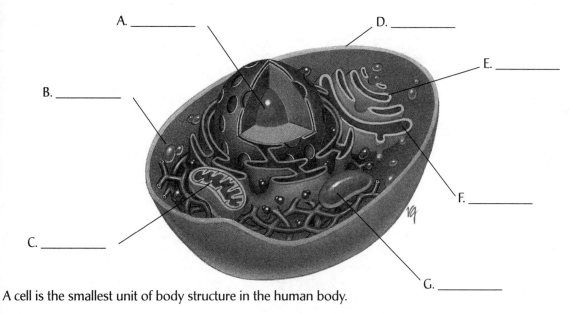

A. _____

B. _____

C. _____

D. _____

E. _____

F. _____

G. _____

A cell is the smallest unit of body structure in the human body.

Figure 8–1

TABLE 8–1

	Cell Part	Function
1.	_____	_____
2.	_____	_____
3.	_____	_____
4.	_____	_____
5.	_____	_____
6.	_____	_____
7.	_____	_____

Identifying Body Planes

Use Figure 8-4 in the textbook to label the diagram of the body planes in Figure 8-2.

1. _____

2. _____

3. _____

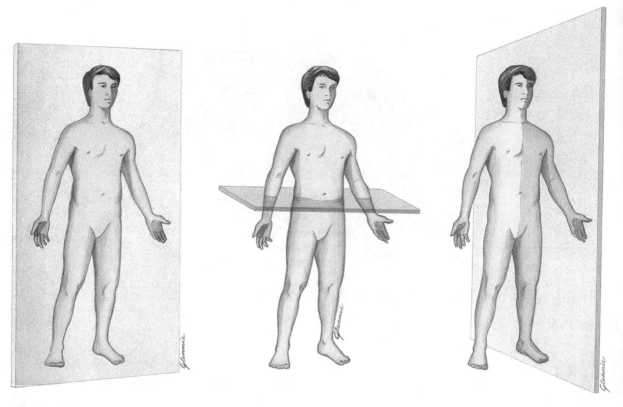

Figure 8–2

Identifying Body Cavities

Use Figure 8-5 in the textbook to label the diagram of the body cavities in Figure 8-3. Shade the cavities that are considered to be located on the dorsal side of the body. In the spaces provided in Table 8-2, list at least two organs or structures found in each body cavity.

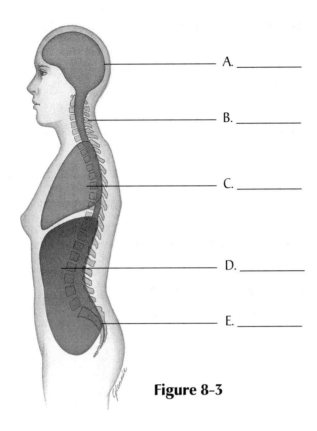

A. _____

B. _____

C. _____

D. _____

E. _____

Figure 8-3

TABLE 8-2

Body Cavity	Structures Located in the Cavity
1. _____	_____
2. _____	_____
3. _____	_____
4. _____	_____
5. _____	_____

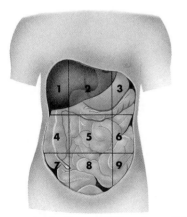

Identifying Body Regions

Use Figure 8-6 in the textbook to label the diagram of the body regions in Figure 8-4.

1. _____

2. _____

3. _____

4. _____

5. _____

6. _____

7. _____

8. _____

9. _____

Figure 8-4 (From Thibodeau GA, Patton KT: Anatomy & Physiology, ed 5, St. Louis, 2003, Mosby)

Identifying Disorders of Body Organization

Complete the missing information about genetic disorders in Table 8-3 using the chapters indicated. Note the etiology (causing factor), signs and symptoms, and treatment and method of prevention (if any). The textbook chapter where information may be found is indicated in parentheses.

Applying Your Knowledge

1. Why is a hereditary characteristic referred to as a condition, syndrome, or disorder instead of a disease?

   _____

   _____

   _____

2. The hereditary condition that affects the appearance of the mouth and that can be corrected with plastic surgery is called _____.

3. The condition that may result in myelomeningocele is called _____.

4. The condition that results in too many red blood cells is called _____.

TABLE 8-3

Disorder	Etiology	Signs and Symptoms	Treatment and Prevention
Cleft lip or palate Chapter 9			
Clubfoot Chapter 13			
Cystic fibrosis Chapter 12			
Down syndrome Chapter 18			
Huntington's chorea Chapter 18			
Klinefelter's syndrome Chapter 20			
Neural tube defect Chapter 18			
Neurofibromatosis Chapter 18			
Phenylketonuria Chapter 15			
Sickle cell anemia Chapter 11			
Tay-Sachs Chapter 15			
Thalassemia Chapter 11			

Investigations

Identifying Tissue Types

Read all directions before beginning the activity. Laboratory activities should be performed only under the supervision of a qualified professional.

Equipment and Supplies
cover slip (optional)
microscope
prepared slides of tissue types
raw chicken wing, blood sample, cheek cells (optional)
slide (optional)

Directions

1. Review the procedure for using a microscope found in Chapter 21.

2. Observe prepared slides of four types of body tissue under low and high power.

3. Draw your observations of the four tissue types in the spaces provided in Figure 8-5.

4. Prepare a wet slide using a thin slide of tissue from a raw chicken wing, cheek cells, blood, or other specimen.

5. Identify the tissue type of the slide.

6. Draw your observation in the space provided in Figure 8-5.

7. Return all equipment and supplies to the designated location.

Drawing Conclusions

1. In your opinion, which kind of tissue is the easiest to identify? Why?

   _____

   _____

   _____

2. Which kind of tissue(s) did you observe in the chicken wing sample?

   _____

   _____

   _____

3. In your opinion, which tissue type is the most diverse or has the most varied structures in the body?

   _____

   _____

   _____

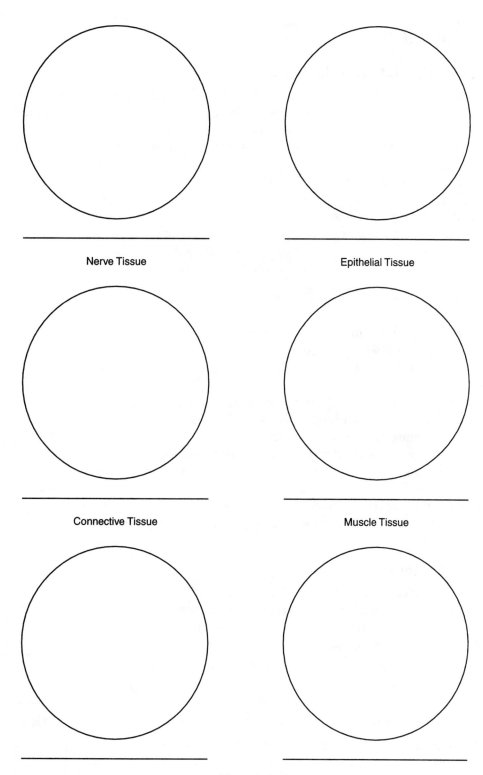

Nerve Tissue   Epithelial Tissue

Connective Tissue   Muscle Tissue

Figure 8-5

Critical Thinking

Determining Probability of Inheritance

Cystic fibrosis is often used to study inherited traits because it is carried by a recessive, nonsexual or autosomal gene. Cystic fibrosis results in inadequate production of certain enzymes. The condition is characterized by excessive mucus in the lungs. It can be detected by testing for salt on the skin. Treatment includes eating a diet that is high in protein and calories. The person with this condition also must use good pulmonary hygiene, which may include postural drainage, to keep the lungs free of excess secretions. Postural drainage involves positioning the body to drain secretions into the bronchi so they may be excreted by coughing. Antibiotics are used to treat infections if they occur. People with cystic fibrosis may live well past middle age with proper care.

Cystic fibrosis is the most commonly occurring recessive disorder in the white population.

The probability of inheriting a genetic disorder may be determined using a Punnet square. In the example of cystic fibrosis, the parents may have a genetic configuration of genotype as follows:

FATHER'S GENOTYPE	MOTHER'S GENOTYPE
Ff	Ff

Both parents are carriers. That means that they both carry the recessive gene (f) for cystic fibrosis, but do not have the condition themselves because it is recessive. Having the dominant gene (F) means that the phenotype or appearance of each of these individuals is not to have cystic fibrosis.

During meiosis, or sexual cell reproduction, the sperm and egg of the mother and father are formed using one of the genes possible for this trait. The chances of the sperm and egg containing the F or the f is exactly equal.

The Punnet square can be used to determine the probability of the offspring to show the condition of cystic fibrosis. It is formed by placing the father's genes on top and the mother's genes on the side as shown in Figure 8-6.

The probability of the offspring having the condition of cystic fibrosis (genotype ff) is one in four or 1/4. The probability of the offspring being a carrier (genotype Ff) is two in four or 1/2.

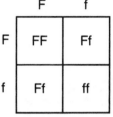

	F	f
F	FF	Ff
f	Ff	ff

Figure 8-6

Examining the Evidence

1. Complete the Punnet square in Figure 8-7 to determine the probability of a couple showing the following genotypes producing an offspring with cystic fibrosis. The father's phenotype is that he has the condition (genotype = ff). The mother is a carrier (genotype = Ff).

    The probability of the offspring having cystic fibrosis (genotype ff) is _____ in four or _____. The probability of the offspring being a carrier (genotype Ff) is _____ in four or _____. The probability of the couple producing a child without the condition is _____ in four or _____.

	f	f
F		
f		

Figure 8-7

2. Complete the punnet square in Figure 8-8 for a couple who have the following phenotypes. The father is a carrier (genotype = _____). The mother does not carry this recessive gene (genotype = _____).

    The probability of the offspring having cystic fibrosis (genotype ff) is _____ in four or _____. The probability of the offspring being a carrier (genotype Ff) is _____ in four or _____. The probability of the couple producing a child without the condition is _____ in four or _____.

Figure 8-8

3. Why is the probability of the second child showing the condition of cystic fibrosis for the couple in question #1 the same as the probability of their first child having this genetic configuration?

_____

_____

_____

4. Why is the probability of the sperm containing the F or f gene exactly the same when the father's genotype is Ff?

_____

_____

_____

9 *Integumentary System*

Vapid Vocabulary

Before reading the chapter, challenge your knowledge of words used in the chapter by completing the crossword puzzle of glossary terms.

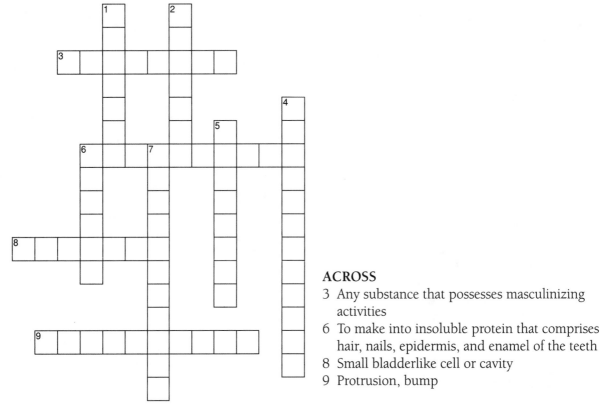

ACROSS

3 Any substance that possesses masculinizing activities
6 To make into insoluble protein that comprises hair, nails, epidermis, and enamel of the teeth
8 Small bladderlike cell or cavity
9 Protrusion, bump

DOWN

1 To supply water to in order to restore or maintain fluid balance
2 Organic material that gives color in the body
4 Removal of hair using electricity
5 Loss of appetite; eating disorder
6 Sharply elevated, irregularly shaped scar that progressively enlarges
7 Period of growth from appearance of secondary gender characteristics to cessation of body (somatic) growth; roughly 12 to 18 years of age

Key Search

Find the Key Terms from the chapter in the word search puzzle below. Define each of the terms in the space provided.

```
N  P  W  X  X  L  O  R  P  P  S  V  F  M  F  G  N  D  A  D  S  L  I  D  C
S  I  M  R  E  D  I  P  E  A  N  U  H  I  T  A  E  Z  B  P  V  R  E  T  I
G  S  Q  O  G  V  F  D  V  H  P  G  O  T  W  R  T  R  O  N  X  R  G  B  V
X  R  U  V  M  B  Z  S  R  D  A  I  Y  E  M  I  Q  J  P  O  M  M  I  N  L
W  I  I  L  W  L  L  O  S  T  H  E  L  I  C  M  R  B  O  A  V  P  T  G  O
I  A  J  W  I  P  R  C  U  S  A  L  S  L  W  A  I  A  T  G  C  R  Y  N  F
S  A  H  U  Z  P  D  P  A  D  J  A  P  D  A  Q  B  I  V  N  K  E  X  G  B
V  U  T  L  J  M  K  Z  O  N  R  J  A  J  N  W  T  E  X  G  S  P  L  T  X
F  K  D  V  I  K  Q  Z  H  H  S  O  O  Y  T  I  V  R  S  O  X  Y  G  Z  S
W  P  P  O  A  R  N  F  H  U  I  L  W  O  S  Z  A  V  P  P  H  Z  P  T  P
X  N  E  J  R  X  R  M  J  K  D  P  T  I  H  J  S  I  S  O  T  G  E  D  D
B  E  G  W  X  I  W  O  A  E  U  T  T  N  O  K  D  H  Y  S  D  R  A  Y  D
Q  M  R  Q  N  A  F  O  U  V  C  Q  Y  O  L  A  I  A  F  K  C  Y  S  V  A
X  A  Z  U  B  H  X  E  W  J  C  X  B  U  G  F  Z  E  P  G  E  I  E  W  J
U  R  X  G  T  K  F  U  R  S  Y  I  O  O  E  C  P  L  A  N  R  K  Z  S  I
B  J  V  J  C  H  E  G  Z  O  G  S  J  U  U  E  Q  C  J  B  K  Z  B  J  W
M  E  L  A  N  I  N  S  Y  U  U  T  V  G  X  R  H  I  S  I  O  O  D  Y  N
V  A  L  B  L  Z  Q  K  V  N  A  S  R  E  L  U  W  L  L  O  X  H  K  V  C
X  W  N  S  U  B  C  U  T  A  N  E  O  U  S  M  V  L  H  P  E  M  S  Q  O
L  W  Q  S  W  Z  B  A  I  X  T  Y  T  A  L  I  B  O  H  S  I  G  T  C  M
F  S  S  G  E  J  L  C  S  R  A  D  P  D  O  N  F  F  K  Y  X  X  I  E  R
V  G  P  A  Y  L  K  S  R  D  W  V  G  X  N  O  J  I  Z  N  X  R  N  Q  R
A  K  D  X  M  X  J  E  T  D  B  I  X  A  L  U  J  M  K  Y  V  N  P  A  E
A  L  U  N  U  L  A  R  E  R  T  T  I  L  E  S  V  K  M  N  K  B  N  L  Y
Z  M  N  V  Z  T  L  O  R  D  X  C  I  U  L  K  X  P  T  P  J  K  W  T  J
```

1. Adipose- _____

2. Biopsy-_____

3. Ceruminous- _____

4. Dermatitis-_____

5. Dermis- _____

6. Epidermis-_____

7. Follicle- _____

8. Lunula- _____

9. Melanin- _____

10. Papilla-_____

11. Pilus- _____

12. Sebaceous-_____

13. Subcutaneous-_____

14. Sudoriferous-_____

Just the Facts

1. The skin is the _ _ _ _ _ _ _ _ _ _ _ _ _ in the body.

2. The three types of glands in the skin are the _ _ _ _ _ _ _ _ _ _ glands,
   _ _ _ _ _ _ _ _ _ _ _ _ glands, and the
   _ ⃝ _ _ _ _ _ _ _ _ _ glands.

3. Ceruminous glands are located only in the _ _ _ ⃝ _ _ _ _ _ _ _ _ _ _
   of the ear.

4. Skin disorders are usually uncomfortable and unattractive but not
   _ _ _ _ _-_ _ _ _ _ _ _ _ _ _ _ _ _.

5. Acne usually appears in adolescence and often is caused by the
   _ _ _ ⃝ _ _ _ _ _ _ _ _ _ _ _ _ _ _ _ _ of oil related to
   increased hormones during puberty.

6. Two skin disorders that lead to a change in pigmentation include _ _ _ _ _ _ _ _
   and _ _ _ _ _ _ _ _.

7. Two skin disorders caused by bacteria include _ _ _ _ _ _ _ _ _ _ and
   _ ⃝ _ _ _ _ _ _.

8. All soaps work by emulsification; they surround and bind to the dirt so that it can be
   _ _ _ _ _ ⃝ _ _ _.

9. The skin defends against the damaging ultraviolet radiation of the sun by producing
   _ _ _ _ _ _ _.

10. _ _ ⃝ _ _ _ _ _ _ carcinoma is the most common type of skin cancer.

Use the circled letters to form the answer to this jumble. Clue: What is the layer of the skin that contains the blood and nerve vessels called?

— — — — — —

Concept Applications

Identifying Structures of the Cell

Use Figure 9-1 in the textbook to label the diagram of the skin in Figure 9-1. Describe the function of each part in Table 9-1.

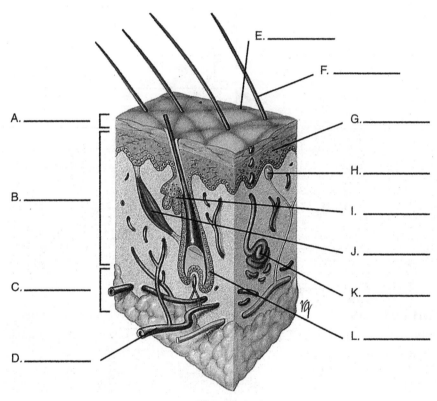

E. _____

F. _____

A. _____

G. _____

H. _____

B. _____

I. _____

J. _____

C. _____

K. _____

D. _____

L. _____

Figure 9-1

TABLE 9-1   **Skin Parts and Their Function**

Skin Part	Main Function
Epidermis	
Dermis	
Subcutaneous	
Hair shaft	
Pore	
Melanocyte	
Nerve cell	
Sebaceous gland	
Arrector pili	
Hair root	
Sudoriferous gland	
Blood vessel	

Identifying Skin Lesions

Use the descriptions of skin lesions in Table 9-2 in the textbook to identify the diagrams. Identify the possible cause in Table 9-2 on p. 95.

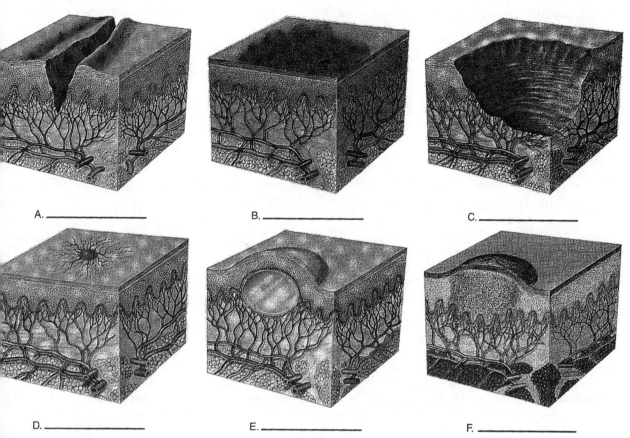

A. _____ B. _____ C. _____

D. _____ E. _____ F. _____

Figure 9-2 A, Courtesy of Thompson JM et al: *Mosby's Clinical Nursing,* ed 3, St. Louis, 1993, Mosby–Year Book, Inc.; B, Courtesy of Seidel: *Mosby's Guide to Physical Examination,* ed 3, St. Louis, 1995, Mosby–Year Book, Inc.; C, Courtesy of Thompson JM et al: *Mosby's Clinical Nursing,* ed 3, St. Louis, 1993, Mosby–Year Book, Inc.; D, Courtesy of Seidel: *Mosby's Guide to Physical Examination,* ed 3, St. Louis, 1995, Mosby–Year Book, Inc.; E-F, Courtesy of Thompson JM et al: *Mosby's Clinical Nursing,* ed 3, St. Louis, 1993, Mosby–Year Book, Inc.

TABLE 9-2   Skin Lesions and Their Causes

Lesion	Cause
Fissure	
Ulcer	
Cyst	
Papule	

Applying Your Knowledge

1. The hereditary condition that results in a shortage of melanocytes in the skin is called

_____. One of the problems that may result from this condition is

damage to the vision because _____ _____

_____ _____.

2. One fungal condition of the skin that may occur in people using the same gym area is called

_____ _____

3. A preventable sore of the skin and underlying tissues resulting from pressure is called a

_____ _____ .

4. A very contagious bacterial infection of the skin that is common in children is called

_____ .

5. The three forms of skin cancer are _____ , _____ , and

_____ . The most serious form is _____ . A fourth form,

Karposi's sarcoma, has become associated with the infection commonly called

_____ .

Identifying Disorders of the Integumentary System

Use the textbook to complete the missing information about integumentary system disorders in Table 9-3 of the textbook. Note the name of the disorder, etiology (causing factor), signs and symptoms, and treatment and method of prevention (if any) where missing.

TABLE 9-3

Disorder	Etiology (cause)	Signs and Symptoms	Treatment and Prevention
			Antibiotics and isolation to prevent spread of disease
	Increased secretion of oil due to increased hormone section		
		Three forms; lesions; spot or growth that does not heal	
		Skin blisters; itching; cracks; especially between the toes	
	Prolonged pressure and hypoxia to affected tissues		
		Itching of the scalp; white flakes	
	Virus	Papule, plantar may disappear	

Applying Standard and Transmission-Based Isolation Precautions

The Communicable Disease Center has established special procedures such as wearing gloves, masks, and gowns to prevent the spread of infection. The procedures used depend on the method by which the pathogen is spread. In 1987, universal body substance isolation precautions were developed and recommended for use with all clients. These precautions require that the health care worker provide barriers between the blood and body fluids of the client and all others. Chapter 3 in the textbook provides further information regarding universal precautions.

Blood-borne pathogen guidelines were developed to control the spread of hepatitis.

Examining theEvidence

1. On which individual or individuals in the health care setting does the responsibility for following universal precautions fall?

   _____

   _____

   _____

2. Before the use of universal precautions, how could an infectoin have been spread throughout the health care facility before it was diagnosed?

   _____

   _____

   _____

3. Hepatitis A is a virus spread by the fecal-oral route. Describe a chain of events that might take this bacterium from a client in one room to a client in another room.

   _____

   _____

   _____

4. What are some measures used by public health care providers and community leaders to prevent the spread of hepatitis A?

   _____

   _____

   _____

10 Cardiovascular System

Vapid Vocabulary

Before reading the chapter, challenge your knowledge of words used in the chapter by completing the crossword puzzle of glossary terms.

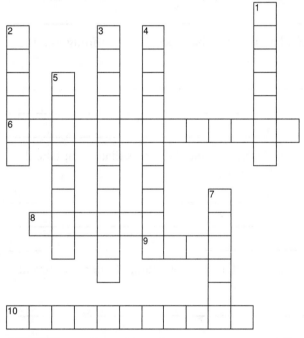

ACROSS

6 Substance preventing the coagulation or clotting of blood
8 Not malignant or cancerous, not recurring
9 Tube for passage of excretions or secretions
10 Act of depriving of oxygen

DOWN

1 Chemical substance produced in the body that has specific regulatory effects on the activity of a certain organ
2 Pertaining to a wall separating two cavities such as in the nose or in the heart
3 Narrowing of a vessel
4 Mechanical radiant energy, sound waves beyond the range of the human ear
5 Tube for injecting or removing a fluid from a cavity such as the bladder or heart
7 Wide opening such as in the ductus arteriosus in the heart

Key Search

Find the Key Terms from the chapter in the word search puzzle below. Define each of the terms in the space provided.

```
N  A  P  T  S  E  M  C  D  E  P  E  C  E  P  N  Y  N  N  P
E  O  S  U  G  I  O  N  E  M  P  I  O  N  M  N  R  M  N  F
R  L  I  O  L  R  S  E  L  O  D  D  N  H  S  O  A  E  S  E
X  R  I  S  O  M  N  O  C  M  E  I  T  D  R  I  T  N  A  G
I  I  A  N  R  E  O  S  N  T  H  Y  R  O  E  T  E  S  I  O
A  A  A  O  R  E  O  N  A  E  H  N  A  P  R  A  M  E  A  I
L  R  I  T  E  H  V  V  A  R  T  R  C  O  E  L  S  L  T  E
Y  T  R  M  T  E  E  O  E  R  A  S  T  O  T  U  Y  I  H  S
N  R  Y  E  E  N  I  N  I  S  Y  M  Y  F  C  C  M  N  M  I
R  M  T  C  E  H  E  E  S  D  S  A  Y  E  A  R  E  E  Y  N
E  S  E  L  O  T  S  A  I  D  R  E  E  C  F  I  R  S  E  G
S  Y  S  T  O  L  E  S  L  E  G  A  L  I  I  C  E  I  L  E
I  R  A  E  E  T  Y  S  I  I  I  E  C  M  R  R  P  E  O  M
O  E  A  I  N  F  A  R  C  T  I  O  N  E  O  E  Y  I  G  E
R  A  A  E  O  R  E  I  I  N  R  M  E  T  E  R  E  F  R  X
A  E  R  L  A  I  N  A  R  C  A  R  T  S  I  R  O  A  A  N
P  O  L  Y  N  E  U  R  I  T  I  S  I  Y  E  Y  E  N  P  E
I  T  U  L  O  A  F  N  I  A  E  R  A  S  E  E  S  C  H  E
G  N  I  N  N  L  N  H  H  E  E  E  X  I  A  E  M  E  Y  E
A  A  R  T  E  E  E  O  U  R  E  T  D  E  E  A  T  E  E  E
```

1. Cardioversion-_____

2. Contract- _____

3. Coronary- _____

4. Diastole- _____

5. Infarction- _____

6. Pulmonary (circulation)-_____

7. Rate- _____

8. Rhythm- _____

9. Stenosis- _____

10. Stethoscope- _____

11. Systemic (circulation)-_____

12. Systole- _____

Just the Facts

1. The structures of the cardiovascular system are the _ _ _ _ _ and the
   _ _ ◯ _ _ _ _ _ _ _ _ _ _ _.

2. _ _ _ _ ◯ _ _ _ circulation refers to the path of the blood from the intestines, gallbladder, pancreas, stomach, and spleen through the liver.

3. The heart has four chambers called _ _ ◯ _ _ and
   _ _ _ _ _ _ _ _ _ _ _.

4. Three main types of blood vessels are _ _ _ _ _ _ _ _, veins, and
   _ _ _ _ _ _ _ _ _ _ _.

5. There are _ _ _ _ _ body locations where the pulse can be counted.

6. Blood _ _ _ _ _ _ ◯ _ is the force of the blood against the walls of the
   _ _ _ _ _ _ _ _.

7. The "lub-dup" sound of the heart results from the opening and closing of the
   _ _ _ _ _ _.

8. The pattern of electrical activity in heart contractions can be measured graphically with an
   _ ◯ _ _ _ _ _ _ _ _ _ _ _ _ _ _ _.

9. Three cardiovascular system disorders that may be treated with a change in diet are atherosclero-
   sis, _ _ _ _ _ _ _ _ _ _ _ ◯ , and
   ◯ _ _ _ _ _ _ _ _ _ _ _ _ _ _ _ _ _ _.

10. Cardiac arrhythmia is a disturbance of the heart's _ _ ◯ _ _ _ caused by a defect in
    the heart's ◯ _ _ _ _ _ _ _ _ cells or by damage to heart tissue.

Use the circled letters to form the answer to this jumble. Clue: What is the circulation called when it travels from the heart to the lungs and back?

— _ _ _ _ _ _ _ _ _ _

Concept Applications

Identifying Structures of the Heart

Use Figure 10-2 in the textbook to label the diagram of the heart in Figure 10-1. In the spaces provided in Table 10-1, indicate whether the blood in each of the structures is oxygenated or deoxygenated. Indicate where the blood will go when it leaves each structure listed.

The human adult heart beats 10,000 times a day.

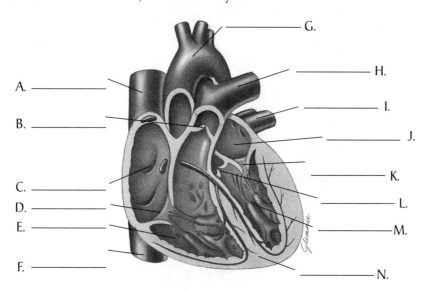

Figure 10-1

TABLE 10-1   HEART STRUCTURE

Structure	Oxygenated (O) or Deoxygenated (D)	Blood Goes from Here to the . . .
1.		
2.		
3.		
4.		
5.		
6.		
7.		
8.		
9.		
10.		
11.		
12.		
13.		
14.		

Identifying Blood Vessels

Use Figure 10-4 in the textbook to label the blood vessels in Figure 10-2. Shade the portion of the diagram that indicates deoxygenated blood.

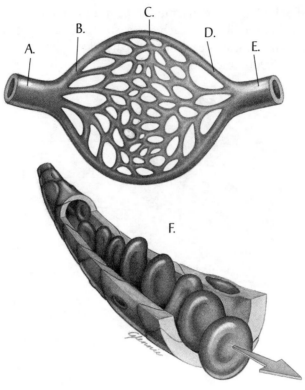

Figure 10-2

A. _____   D. _____

B. _____   E. _____

C. _____   F. _____

Identifying Principal Arteries and Veins

Use Figure 10-5 in the textbook to label the principal arteries and veins in Figure 10-3. Indicate the eight arteries commonly used to measure a pulse rate with an asterisk (*).

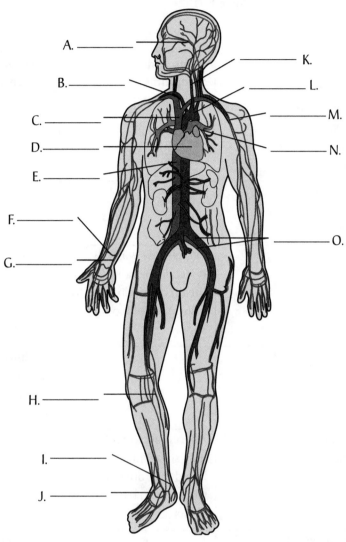

Figure 10-3 Courtesy of Sorrentino: *Mosby's Textbook for Nursing Assistants*, ed 5, Hanover, 2000, Mosby Lifeline

A. _____	F. _____	K. _____
B. _____	G. _____	L. _____
C. _____	H. _____	M. _____
D. _____	I. _____	N. _____
E. _____	J. _____	O. _____

Identifying Disorders of the Cardiovascular System

Complete the table of cardiovascular disorders in Table 10-2 using information provided in Chapter 10 of the textbook. Note the name of the disorder, etiology (causing factor), signs and symptoms, and treatment and method of prevention (if any) where missing.

TABLE 10-2

Disorder	Etiology	Signs and Symptoms	Treatment and Prevention
	Defect in heart's pacemaker or damage to heart tissue		
	Bacterial infection that begins in the throat		
		Vessels lose elasticity resulting in shortness of breath or fainting due to a shortage of blood supply	
			Treatment may include surgery to clear blocked coronary arteries or drugs to dissolve clots
	May be congenital	Abnormal blood flow may sometimes be heard over area of weakness in blood vessel	
	Prolonged sitting or standing		Surgical removal of clotted veins or dissolving drugs
		Veins enlarged and ineffective leading to swelling, bluish veins, redness, and pain	

Applying Your Knowledge

1. The disorder that results in damage to the heart muscle is called _____.

2. One of the complications that may result from _____ is the development of an embolus.

3. In some cases, the sound of abnormal blood flow may be heard in the condition called an

   _____.

4. The condition that results in more than 50% of the deaths in the United States each yeasr is called

   _____   _____.

5. The condition that commonly occurs in people who stand for long periods is called

   _____.

Critical Thinking

Interpreting Electrocardiographs

Using the ECG pattern in Figure 10-4, answer the following questions regarding the tracing.

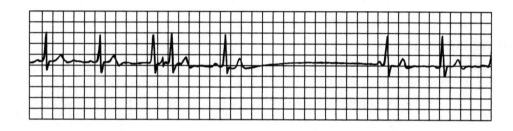

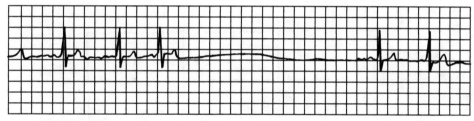

Figure 10-4

Examining the Evidence

1. What kind of heart activity does this ECG pattern represent?

   _____

   _____

   _____

2. Why would or would not this condition be life threatening?

   _____

   _____

   _____

3. What is the objective of treatment for a person with this ECG pattern?

_____

_____

_____

4. Why are ECG studies often performed with the person exercising, such as in a treadmill study?

_____

_____

_____

5. Why would it be necessary to perform a continuous ECG study using a portable monitor with a log of activities? Give at least two reasons.

_____

_____

_____

Calculating Heart Rates

The ECG pattern can also be used to calculate the heart rate. The tracing is made on grid paper that progresses at a standard recording rate of 25 mm/sec. Figure 10-5 illustrates the time requried to record in each of the boxes of the ECG grid paper. To determine the rate, count the number of small boxes and multiply by 0.04 second.

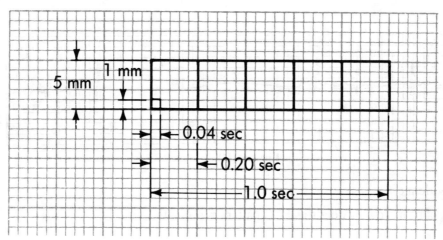

Figure 10-5 Courtesy of Grauer: *A Practical Guide to ECG Interpretation*, ed 2, St. Louis 1998, Mosby.

Calculate the heart rate for each of the illustrated ECG patterns in Figure 10-6A and B.

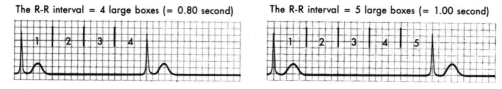

Figure 10-6 Courtesy of Grauer: *A Practical Guide to ECG Interpretation*, ed 2, St. Louis 1998, Mosby.

Calculate the time interval between each of the heart beats in the ECG pattern in Figure 10-7.

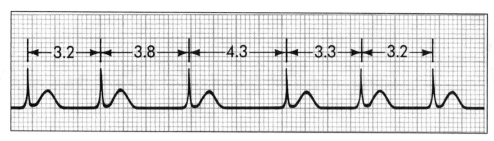

Figure 10-7 Courtesy of Grauer: *A Practical Guide to ECG Interpretation,* ed 2, St. Louis 1998, Mosby.

Examining the Evidence

1. The rate of the heart described in Figure 10-6A is _____ beats per minute.

2. The rate of the heart described in Figure 10-6B is _____ beats per minute.

3. If the heart is regular, the rate can be determined by dividing 300 by the number of large boxes in the R-R interval. Why is this true?

   _____

   _____

   _____

4. By how many seconds would you multiply the R-R interval measurement if you counted the boxes that are 5 mm instead of the smallest that are 1 mm in length?

   _____

   _____

   _____

5. Draw an ECG that shows a rate of 100 beats per minute on the grid paper in Figure 10-8.

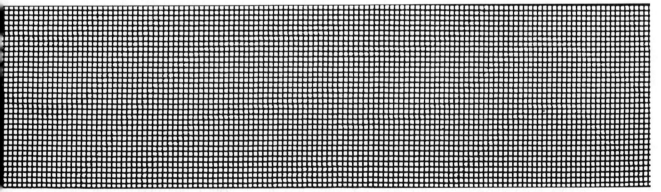

Figure 10-8

11 Circulatory System

Vapid Vocabulary

Before reading the chapter, challenge your knowledge of words used in the chapter by completing the crossword puzzle of glossary terms.

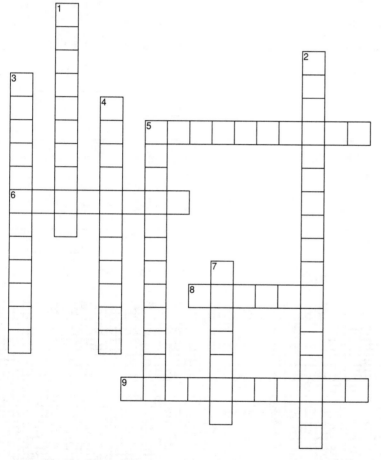

ACROSS

5 Machine that separates lighter portions of a solution, mixture, or suspension by centrifugal force
6 Group of signs and symptoms that characterize a condition or disease
8 Lack of color, paleness
9 Disturbance, impairment, or abnormality in functioning of an organ

DOWN

1 Directed against the body's own tissue
2 Prevention or diminution of immune response

3 Placed between, usually referring to between tissues
4 Enlargement or overgrowth of an organ or part caused by an increase in its cells
5 Treatment of disease by chemical agent
7 Increased discomfort and decreased efficiency caused by prolonged or excessive exertion; exhaustion

Key Search

Find the Key Terms from the chapter in the word search puzzle below. Define each of the terms in the space provided.

```
T  E  P  L  A  S  M  A  J  W  X  Y  A  H  C  T  L  C  B  S
U  M  S  N  F  U  N  P  F  T  A  R  A  W  E  H  K  M  M  O
N  E  G  R  E  L  L  A  X  I  K  T  Y  U  V  R  C  I  X  A
B  Y  P  M  E  K  F  U  M  Z  Y  E  Y  D  N  O  Y  V  P  I
V  L  M  B  W  R  V  E  A  C  V  M  W  O  O  M  M  H  A  M
S  P  J  R  G  I  N  D  O  Z  H  O  I  J  Y  B  Z  B  U  V
G  E  T  Q  E  A  T  F  S  J  R  T  G  Q  S  O  I  W  H  Q
P  T  R  M  A  R  W  B  L  U  A  O  W  B  K  C  Y  T  L  Q
B  K  D  U  M  B  Y  X  N  M  B  H  I  J  D  Y  D  K  N  I
G  I  U  V  M  C  B  T  M  A  D  P  K  N  P  T  N  A  M  A
K  E  Y  J  G  O  K  A  H  Q  R  O  U  L  O  E  B  O  O  L
Y  X  D  Q  K  N  L  N  G  R  S  R  R  A  X  J  X  B  E  Y
B  P  P  C  T  F  K  U  Z  A  O  T  A  V  L  H  O  U  N  T
V  B  U  L  N  D  V  M  Q  I  K  C  N  E  S  H  K  W  N  I
X  I  E  I  R  R  T  A  U  G  J  E  Y  L  C  O  X  Y  J  N
C  O  A  G  U  L  A  T  I  O  N  P  V  T  C  R  Z  N  R  U
I  R  T  H  S  B  H  D  G  L  H  S  P  Y  E  Q  H  Z  F  M
Z  X  O  K  X  W  S  E  F  I  F  F  T  Q  U  W  G  S  C  M
O  R  G  N  S  G  Q  H  X  H  T  E  I  V  Z  Z  C  F  V  I
L  X  O  S  K  I  L  U  H  X  Q  V  K  A  E  X  L  G  Q  D
```

1. Allergen- _____

2. Anemia- _____

3. Antibody- _____

4. Coagulation- _____

5. Erythrocyte- _____

6. Immunity- _____

7. Inflammation- _____

8. Leukocyte-_____

9. Plasma- _____

10. Serum-_____

11. Spectrophotometry- _____

12. Thrombocyte- _____

Just the Facts

1. _ _ _ Ⓞ _ _ _ _ _ _ is the study of blood.

2. Erythrocytes contain a protein called _ _ _ _ _ Ⓞ _ _ _ _ that carries oxygen to all cells and removes carbon dioxide.

3. _ _ _ _ Ⓞ _ _ _ _ _ fight disease and infection.

4. Platelets, also called _ _ _ _ _ _ Ⓞ _ _ _ _ _, promote clotting to prevent blood loss.

5. Type AB blood is called the _ _ _ Ⓞ _ Ⓞ _ _ _ recipient because it has no _ Ⓞ _ _ _ _ _ _ _ _ in the plasma to react with other blood cells.

6. Lymph has two important functions including maintenance of the _ _ Ⓞ _ ' _ fluid _ _ _ _ _ _ Ⓞ and providing immunity.

7. Three disorders of the circulatory system that are forms of cancer are Hodgkin's disease, _ _ _ _ _ _ _ _ _, and _ _ _ _ _ _ _ _ _ Ⓞ _ _ _ _.

8. Two disorders of the circulatory system that are genetic are _ _ _ _ _ _ _ _ _ Ⓞ _ and sickle cell _ Ⓞ _ _ _ _.

9. _ Ⓞ _ _ _ _ _ _ _ _ transfusion is the collection and transfusion of a person's own blood.

10. _ _ _ _ _ _ _ _ Ⓞ may be donated through a process called apheresis.

Use the circled letters to form the answer to this jumble. Clue: What is the person that can donate blood to all people called?

_ _ _ _ _ _ _ _ _ _ _ _ _ _ _

Concept Applications

Identifying Hematocrit Values

Use Figure 11-1 in the textbook to label the diagram of a hematocrit in Figure 11-1. In the spaces provided in Table 11-1, describe the components of each part.

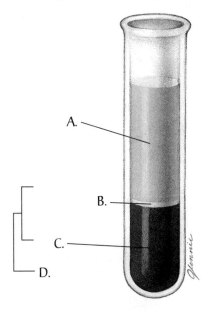

A.

B.

C.

D.

Figure 11-1

TABLE 11-1   BLOOD COMPONENTS

Blood Part	Components
1. _____	_____
	_____
2. _____	_____
	_____

Identifying Formed Elements of Blood

Use Table 11-1 in the textbook to label the diagram of the formed elements of the blood in Figure 11-2. In the spaces provided in Table 11-2, describe the components of each part.

TABLE 11-2   FORMED ELEMENTS

Element	Main Function
1. _____	_____
2. _____	_____
3. _____	_____
4. _____	_____
5. _____	_____
6. _____	_____
7. _____	_____

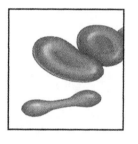

A. _____

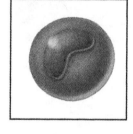

B. _____

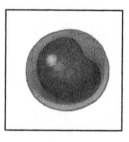

C. _____

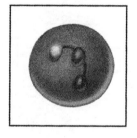

D. _____

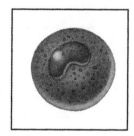

E. _____

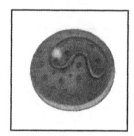

F. _____

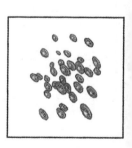

G. _____

Figure 11-2

Determining Blood Compatibility

Table 11-3 indicates the antigens (agglutinogens) found on the red blood cells (RBCs) of the major blood groupings. The plasma of each of the blood groups contains antibodies that react and clot if incompatible antigens are present.

TABLE 11-3

Blood Type	Antigens on RBCs	Antibodies in Plasma
A	A	Anti–B*
B	B	Anti–A†
AB	A & B	none
O	none	Anti-A & Anti-B

*Causes blood to clot if B antigen is present.
†Causes blood to clot if A antigen is present.

Complete Table 11-4 of blood type compatibility indicating whether the blood can be safely transfused from the donor to the recipient by placing a "+" to indicate acceptable transfusion and "−" to indicate that clotting would occur.

TABLE 11-4

	Recipient			
Blood Type	**A**	**B**	**AB**	**O**
A				
B				
AB				
O				

(D O N O R)

Identifying Disorders of the Circulatory System

Use the textbook to complete the missing information about circulatory disorders in Table 11-5. Note the etiology (causing factor), signs and symptoms, and treatment and method of prevention (if any).

TABLE 11–5

Disorder	Etiology	Signs and Symptoms	Treatment and Prevention
	Sex–linked genetic defect of blood coatulation		
		Fatigue, shortness of breath, pallor, rapid heart rate	
	Acute infection such as scarlet fever		
		Painless enlargement of lymph nodes, apears most often in men	
			Elevation of the affected part, anticoagulants, surgery
		Body's immune system turns against itself, Hashimoto's disease is one example	
	Blood cancer		

Applying Your Knowledge

1. Malformed blood cells characterize the inherited blood disorder known as _____ _____ _____.

2. A condition that results in an abnormal increase in the number of red blood cells is called _____.

3. Hodgkin's disease results in cancer of the _____ system and often is found in people _____ to _____ years of age.

4. Myasthenia gravis and systemic lupus are both examples of conditions that are considered to be _____ because the body's cells turn against themselves.

5. Bone marrow transplantation and isolation to prevent infection are just two treatments used for the condition of _____, which is often called _____ _____.

Investigations

Using a Finger Puncture to Type Blood

Determining a person's blood types can be easily performed with a simple finger puncture to obtain a sample of blood. (If it is preferable to use artificial blood, samples are available through several biological supply companies.) Read all directions before beginning the activity. Laboratory activities should be performed only under the supervision of a qualified professional.

Equipment and Supplies

alcohol pledgets or swabs	gloves
A-antiserum	microscope slides
B-antiserum	sterile lancets
Rh-antiserum	toothpicks

Directions

1. Wash your hands thoroughly before beginning this activity. Disposable gloves should be worn by the person performing the puncture to prevent the spread of disease through body secretions.

2. Label and prepare three microscope slides or other designated media with one drop each of A-antiserum, B-antiserum, and Rh-antiserum. These antisera will cause clumping of blood cells when the designated blood protein is mixed with it.

3. With an alcohol swab cleanse the area to be punctured. Either side of the tip of the middle or ring finger can be used for puncture. The area selected should be free from calluses, cuts, and rashes. If the skin feels cool to the touch, soaking the hand to be punctured in warm water will help to increase circulation.

4. The finger to be punctured is held securely while the hand is rested on a solid surface. A sterile lancet is used to pierce the skin in a quick, downward motion. The puncture is made at a right angle to the lines forming the fingerprint.

5. Wipe away the first drop of blood with the alcohol swab because it may be contaminated with skin tissue from the puncture.

6. Place one drop of blood on each of the three designated solutions for blood testing. Do not allow the finger to touch the card or slide containing the antiserum.

7. Hold the alcohol swab on the puncture site until bleeding is stopped.

8. Using a separate toothpick for each slide, stir the blood and antiserum for about 1 minute. Observe for clotting.

9. Record with which of the antisera the blood clotted.

	A-antiserum	B-antiserum	Rh-antiserum
Clotting (Yes/No)	_____	_____	_____
Your blood type is:	_____	_____	_____

Drawing Conclusions

1. If clumping occurs with only A-antiserum, what blood type does that indicate?

_____

_____

_____

2. If no clumping occurs with any of the three antisera, what blood type does that indicate?

_____

_____

_____

3. Why is it important to use three separate toothpicks when mixing the blood with the antiserum?

_____

_____

_____

4. List three possible sources of error in this activity.

_____

_____

_____

Critical Thinking

AIDS Testing

Currently the courts are considering many cases involving individual rights pertaining to testing for diseases and drugs, particularly for HIV (the AIDS virus). In the past, many states required testing for the syphilis bacteria before granting a marriage license. To date, no routine testing program for HIV has been established, although several have been proposed.

Those people who oppose routine testing for HIV fear that testing might lead to discrimination against infected individuals. Additionally, a positive result indicating the presence of the virus without adequate education and counseling might cause serious psychological problems for those tested.

Those people who favor testing feel that the magnitude of the disease cannot be established without a broader base of information. They also believe that those people who come in contact with someone carrying the virus have the right to know.

These issues and the following questions do not have a right or wrong answer. They ask for your opinion based on your personal beliefs. Discussion of these issues may help you to be aware of your own feelings and beliefs.

Examining the Evidence

1. Why would you or would you not support routine testing for HIV?

_____

_____

_____

2. In what situations, if any, would you support the right of a victim of a crime, a health care worker, or an emergency rescue worker to require testing for HIV in someone with whom contact of body secretions has been made?

_____

_____

_____

3. Do you feel that HIV and AIDS are being handled correctly by the Centers for Disease Control and Prevention and other supervising agencies? Explain your answer.

_____

_____

_____

Forensic Serology

Forensic serology is the study of body fluids to provide legal evidence. The pattern of the stain and amount of blood may help determine the activity that occurred during a crime. The blood grouping antigens can be used to help determine to whom the blood belonged.

Examining the Evidence

1. Why can blood typing identification alone be used to exclude certain suspects but cannot be used to determine specifically a person's presence?

_____

_____

_____

2. When a suspect is accused of a crime and blood is found at the scene, explain why you think the officials should or should not have the right to ask for a blood sample.

_____

_____

_____

3. What are at least three criminal situations in which blood or other body secretions may be used as criminal evidence?

_____

_____

_____

12 Respiratory System

Vapid Vocabulary

Before reading the chapter, challenge your knowledge of words used in the chapter by completing the crossword puzzle of glossary terms.

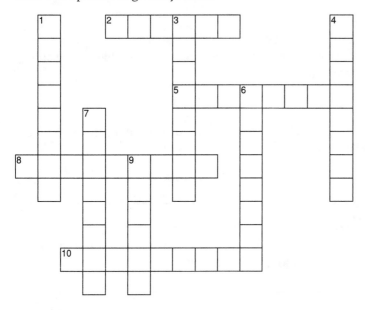

ACROSS

2 Damage
5 Secrete outwardly via a duct
8 Process of being widely spread; spontaneous movement of molecules or other particles in solution to reach uniform concentration
10 Under control of the conscious will

DOWN

1 Pertaining to the chest
3 Chemical-resistant, fibrous mineral form made of magnesium silicate
4 Substance capable of inducing hypersensitive or allergic reaction
6 Holding power
7 Oozing fluids from blood or lymph vessels into body cavities
9 Matter ejected from the respiratory tract through the mouth

Key Search

Find the Key Terms from the chapter in the word search puzzle below. Define each of the terms in the space provided.

K	N	N	W	I	L	Q	M	C	I	T	A	H	R	J
P	C	C	M	J	R	Z	U	Q	K	N	E	Y	P	E
J	P	I	L	N	V	Y	N	O	O	E	N	N	U	O
E	G	R	L	C	O	B	I	I	F	O	P	E	L	M
N	E	X	P	I	R	A	T	I	O	N	U	P	M	D
T	O	G	C	K	A	A	S	T	T	C	E	K	O	X
B	X	I	S	K	R	T	A	I	A	A	N	K	N	V
R	R	P	T	I	I	C	I	N	O	R	H	C	A	Q
R	P	A	P	A	H	A	D	A	P	N	E	A	R	S
S	A	S	D	Y	R	Y	E	M	K	M	O	Z	Y	X
S	E	Y	P	Y	B	I	M	N	G	F	F	J	D	B
R	Z	N	K	F	P	L	P	E	P	B	U	Q	X	X
U	E	Z	V	J	W	N	L	S	T	S	E	R	C	W
A	J	S	P	V	H	H	E	N	N	T	Y	X	Z	O
X	Q	E	X	L	P	O	H	A	D	I	E	D	G	O

1. Apnea- _____

2. Bradypnea- _____

3. Chronic- _____

4. Cilia- _____

5. Dyspnea- _____

6. Eupnea- _____

7. Expiration- _____

8. Inspiration- _____

9. Mediastinum- _____

10. Phlegm- _____

11. Pulmonary- _____

12. Respiration- _____

13. Tachypnea- _____

Just the Facts

1. Both the _ _ _ _ _ ◯ _ _ _ and _ _ _ _ _ _ _ _ _ _ _ _ nervous systems control respiration.

2. The _ _ _ _ _ _ _ are hollow spaces in the bones of the skull that open into the
   nasal cavity.

3. The flap that covers the nasal tract is called the _ _ _ _ _ and the one that covers the
   trachea is called the _ _ _ _ _ ◯ _ _ _ _.

4. Capillaries in the walls of the alveoli exchange oxygen and carbon dioxide by the process of
   _ _ _ _ _ _ _ _ _.

5. The diaphragm _ _ _ _ _ _ _ _ _ and moves downward during inhalation

6. The amount of air that can be brought into the lungs is called
   _ _ _ _ _ _ _ _ _ _ _ _ _ ◯ _ _ _ _ _ _.

7. Chronic obstructive pulmonary disease is a group of chronic respiratory disorders including
   _ _ _ _ _ _, chronic bronchitis, and _ _ _ _ ◯ _ _ _ _ _
   _ _ _ _ _ _ _ _ _ _.

8. Two disorders of the respiratory system that are caused by a virus are
   _ _ _ _ _ _ _ _ _ _ _ and a ◯ _ _ _.

9. One respiratory system disorder that is directly linked to smoking is _ _ _ _
   ◯ _ _ _ _ _.

10. The respiratory disorder that has an increased incidence since 1991 and is the most common
    fatal infectious disease in the world today is _ _ ◯ _ _ _ _ _ _ _ _ _ _.

Use the circled letters to form the answer to this jumble. Clue: What substance is linked to cancer of
the esophagus and ulcers?

_ _ _ _ _ _ _

Concept Applications

Identifying Structures of the Respiratory System

Use Figure 12-1 in the textbook to label the diagram of the respiratory system in Figure 12-1. In the spaces provided in Table 12-1, describe the function of each part.

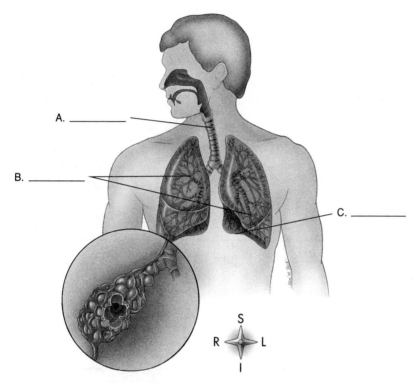

A. _____

B. _____

C. _____

Figure 12-1 Courtesy of Thibodeau GA, Patton KT: *Anatomy and Physiology,* ed 4, St. Louis 1999, Mosby.

TABLE 12-1   FUNCTIONS OF RESPIRATORY SYSTEM STRUCTURES

System Part	Main Function
1. _____	_____
2. _____	_____
3. _____	_____

Reading a Normal Lung Volume

Use Figure 12-3 in the textbook to indicate the correct volume in liters for each of the readings in Figure 12-2. In the spaces provided in Table 12-2, describe what each of the categories represents in relation to breathing.

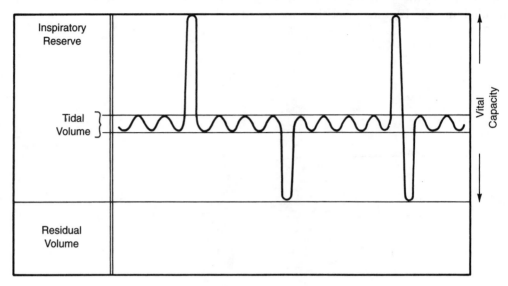

Figure 12-2

TABLE 12-2   LUNG VOLUME READINGS

Lab Reading	What the Reading Represents
1. Residual volume	_____
2. Inspiratory reserve	_____
3. Expiratory reserve	_____
4. Tidal volume	_____
5. Vital capacity	_____

Identifying Disorders of the Respiratory System

Use the textbook to complete the missing information about respiratory disorders in Table 12-3. Note the etiology (causing factor), signs and symptoms, and treatment and method of prevention (if any).

TABLE 12-3

Disorder	Etiology	Signs and Symptoms	Treatment and Prevention
	Caused by one of more than 200 viruses		
		Heavy cough and mucus production leading to thickening of the bronchial walls	
	Upper respiratory infection or changes in atmospheric pressure		
	Virus, bacteria, or chemical or aspiration of fluid	Excessive moisture in the lungs that impairs breathing	
		Affects pharynx, larynx, and nose; may cause loss of voice or hoarseness	
	Bacteria transmitted through the air		
			Surgical removal of lung chemotherapy, and radiation

Applying Your Knowledge

1. An infection that affects the nose, pharynx, or laynx is often called an _____ _____ _____.

2. One of the respiratory system disorders that has increased in incidence and has developed resistance to antibiotics is _____.

3. A buildup of carbon dioxide in the blood can lead to a condition called _____ _____.

4. When air or fluid enters the space around the lungs, it is called _____ _____.

5. A chronic condition in which the alveoli lose their elasticity is called _____.

Investigations

Performing a Lung Volume Reading

The volume of air that is moved in and out of the lung may be used to measure the ability of the body to supply oxygen to the cells. If a wet spirometer is not avaialble for this activity, a large water-filled jar indicating the volume may be substituted, as shown in Figure 12-3. Read all directions before beginning the activity. Laboratory activities should be performed only under the supervision of a qualified professional.

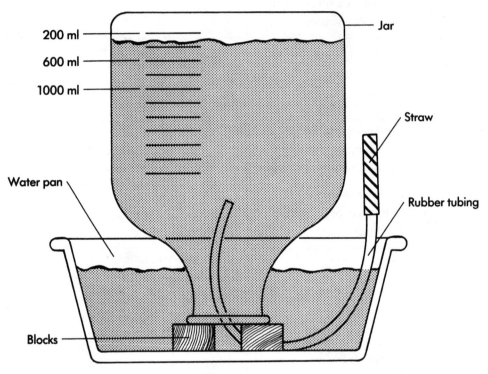

Figure 12-3

Equipment and Supplies

disposable mouthpieces
wet spirometer or jar apparatus

Directions

1. Work in groups of at least two people.

2. Assemble a wet spirometer for lung volume readings. Read the manufacturer's instructions before beginning. Some wet spirometers require INSPIRATION of air instead of EXHALATION as described below. Exhalation is used to measure when the jar apparatus is used.

3. Place a disposable mouthpiece in the breathing tube.

4. Do not look at the gauge during breathing trials. Your partner should read all measurements.

5. To measure the tidal volume, breathe at a normal rate for several minutes. When the normal volume of air for one breath is inhaled through the mouth, gently exhale through the mouthpiece. Perform this measurement three times and compute the average of the resulting volumes.
   Trial #1—_____ liters
   Trial #2—_____ liters   Average = _____ liters
   Trial #3—_____ liters   Tidal Volume

6. To measure your inspiratory reserve, inhale as much air as possible. Breathe the air gently through the mouthpiece until you reach the end of a normal breath. This measurement includes the tidal volume. Perform this measurement three times and compute the average of the resulting volumes.
   Trial #1—_____ liters
   Trial #2—_____ liters   Average = _____ liters
   Trial #3—_____ liters   Inspiratory Reserve + Tidal Volume
   Because the inspiratory reserve that you measured contains the tital volume, you must subtract the average tidal volume from the measured inspiratory reserve to get the true value of the inspiratory reserve.
                         Average = _____ liters
                         True Inspiratory Reserve

7. To measure expiratory reserve, breathe normally several times. After a normal breath has been exhaled, gently blow any remaining air through the mouthpiece. Perform this measurement three times and compute the average of the resulting volumes.
   Trial #1—_____ liters
   Trial #2—_____ liters   Average = _____ liters
   Trial #3—_____ liters   Expiratory Reserve

8. To measure vital capacity, inhale as much air as possible and gently blow through the mouthpiece. Gently exhale as much air as possible through the mouthpiece. Perform this measurement three times and compute the average of the resulting volumes.
   Trial #1—_____ liters
   Trial #2—_____ liters   Average = _____ liters
   Trial #3—_____ liters   Vital Capacity

9. Use a colored pen or pencil to chart your results in Figure 12-4. Compare your results with the normal lung volume reading.

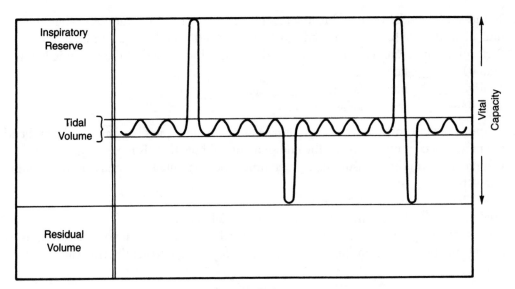

Figure 12-4

Drawing Conclusions

1. Why is the average of three volume measurements used to determine the laboratory results?

   _____

   _____

   _____

2. What is the value of your residual volume? Why can't this value be measured?

   _____

   _____

   _____

3. Vital capacity, by definition, is the sum of the inspiratory reserve, tidal volume, and expiratory reserve. Add these three values as they were measured in the laboratory activity. How does this number compare with the volume of the vital capacity that was measured in the activity? Why may these values differ?

   Inspiratory Reserve + Tidal Volume + Expiratory Reserve = _____

   Measured Vital Capacity = _____

   _____

   _____

   _____

4. Would the vital capacity of an athlete be larger or smaller than someone who does not exercise regularly? Explain your answer.

   _____

   _____

   _____

5. List three possible sources of error in this activity.

_____

_____

_____

Demonstrating the Effect of Smoking on Lung Tissue

Read all directions before beginning the activity. Laboratory activities should be performed only under the supervision of a qualified professional.

Equipment and Supplies

cigarette and match or lighter
cotton balls
irrigation syringe or basting utensil
microscope
microscope slide and cover slip
prepared microscope slide of cancerous lung tissue
prepared microscope slide of normal lung tissue

Directions

1. Place a cigarette in the tip of an irrigation syringe that has been filled loosely with about 1 inch of cotton.

2. "Smoke" the cigarette by pulling air in and out of the syringe using the plunger. NOTE: It is preferable to "smoke" the cigarette outside of the classroom or under a ventilation hood.

3. Prepare a dry mount slide of the cotton after the cigarette has been "smoked."

4. Prepare a dry mount slide of cotton that has not been exposed to the cigarette.

5. Examine the slides under a microscope and compare. Sketch the cotton in the spaces provided in Figure 12-5.

6. Examine slides of normal lung tissue and cancerous tissue. Sketch the tissue in the spaces provided in Figure 12-6.

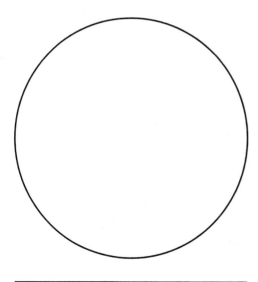 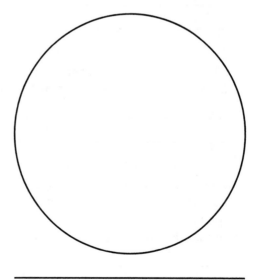

Figure 12-5

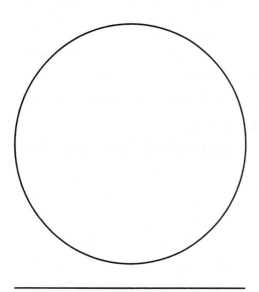
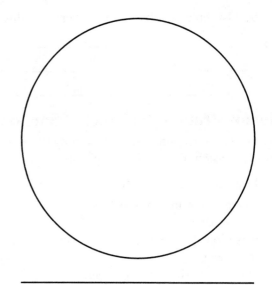

Figure 12-6

Drawing Conclusions

1. What is the residue that can be observed on the cotton after the cigarette smoke has passed through it?

   _____

   _____

   _____

2. How does the normal lung tissue compare with the cancerous tissue in appearance?

   _____

   _____

   _____

3. How might the effect of smoking on the cotton and lung tissue be compared?

   _____

   _____

   _____

4. Why would the high number of blood vessels in the lung tissues make it more likely to suffer damage from cigarettes than another tissue such as the skin?

   _____

   _____

   _____

5. If the current cost of a pack of cigarettes is $2.00, compute the cost of a pack-a-day smoker for 1 year. Assume that this amount of money is placed in an account that earns 7% interest each year. Compute the value of the money in 5 years and 10 years. (HINT: Remember that the amount to be calculated each year should include the interest earned from the prevous year.)

   _____

   _____

   _____

Critical Thinking

Smoking Choices

Rights of the nonsmoker and smoker have become a source of conflict for many people. Laws have been enacted to protect the nonsmoker from "second-hand" smoke by limiting smoking areas and requiring the availability of nonsmoking areas.

Health insurance companies offer lower rates to corporations that offer smoking cessation programs for their employees.

Examining the Evidence

1. Should the rights of nonsmokers be considered more important than those of smokers? Why or why not?

   _____

   _____

   _____

2. Do you believe that a law should be enacted to restrict or eliminate smoking entirely? Explain your answer.

   _____

   _____

   _____

3. With more than 300,000 deaths attributed to smoking each year, why do you think that the number of smokers is actually increasing in some age groups?

   _____

   _____

   _____

4. Most insurance companies give a discount for household policies if the occupants are nonsmokers. They do this because statistics indicate that smokers present a higher risk of fires and other related household claims. Some health insurance companies will not cover expenses due to respiratory illness in smokers. Why would or would you not support this policy?

   _____

   _____

   _____

Changes in Air Pressure

The weight of the air or atmosphere around the earth is approximately 14.7 pounds per square inch (1.03 kg/cm^2). This measurement is defined as one atmosphere of pressure. Atmospheric pressure decreases with increased altitude and increases as a person goes lower than sea level during activities such as scuba diving.

Each 33-foot (10-m) increment of sea water depth increases the pressure one atmosphere. At this depth, the person is under two atmospheres of pressure (one from the air above sea level and one from the pressure of the water).

The primary effect of air pressure for the diver is the volume or density of the air. In a closed container such as a tank or lung, the volume of the air at two atmospheres is reduced due to the increased pressure. This inverse relationship between pressure and volume is called *Boyle's law*. As the volume of the air decreases at greater depths, the diver needs more air to fill his/her lungs.

Boyle's law: At a constant temperature the volume of a gas varies inversely with the pressure exerted on it.

Examining the Evidence

1. How would the volume or density of a liter of air at the top of a mountain compare with the same container of air at sea level?

_____

_____

_____

2. Why might a person who does not usually live at a high altitude become "short of breath" when at a high altitude? What might the person do to correct this situation?

_____

_____

_____

3. Why does the scuba diver need to ascend (go from a deep water level to the water's surface) slowly?

_____

_____

_____

4. What changes in the volume of air in Figure 12-7, showing a closed system descent, occur as the container is taken from sea level to a depth of 66 feet?

_____

_____

_____

5. What changes in the volume of air in Figure 12-8, showing a closed system ascent, occur as the container is taken from a depth of 66 feet to sea level?

_____

_____

_____

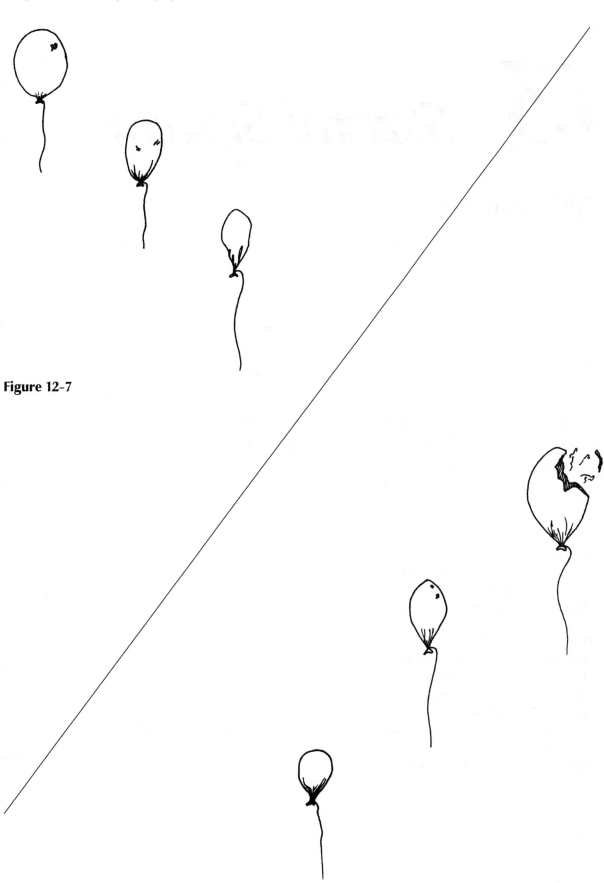

Figure 12-7

Figure 12-8

13 Skeletal System

Vapid Vocabulary

Before reading the chapter, challenge your knowledge of words used in the chapter by completing the crossword puzzle of glossary terms.

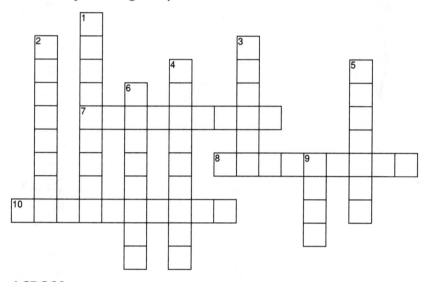

ACROSS

7 Loss or impairment of motor function
8 Having no organs; not derived from hydrocarbons
10 Passed genetically, from one generation to another

DOWN

1 Time of life during which menstruation stops permanently
2 To project through an abnormal opening in the wall of a body cavity
3 Not malignant or cancerous, not recurring
4 Tending to become progressively worse and result in death
5 Pertaining to an organ; having organized structure; chemical substances containing carbon
6 Act of rubbing
9 Swelling of the joints resulting in a buildup of uric acid caused by some metabolic disorder

Key Search

Find the Key Terms from the chapter in the word search puzzle below. Define each of the terms in the space provided.

```
L  G  I  R  T  R  N  T  E  S  O  W  A  N  N  V  I  O  C  L
O  L  E  S  N  N  N  R  U  T  C  O  B  A  R  I  R  Y  L  C
N  E  G  T  E  E  V  O  L  I  A  R  U  R  N  O  I  T  N  M
V  E  I  A  M  I  L  E  D  A  O  R  R  R  T  A  T  C  L  O
O  O  V  A  O  L  T  E  A  T  L  A  S  R  U  G  G  E  S  E
E  C  G  T  E  T  P  I  I  C  G  M  A  A  M  N  E  D  V  L
N  I  A  C  O  O  T  W  M  C  E  D  E  D  O  C  E  I  N  C
L  V  N  R  H  I  E  Y  O  E  E  M  N  L  A  O  T  G  O  M
E  A  O  T  T  C  O  Y  C  W  R  W  L  L  T  A  T  L  I  S
C  L  R  O  I  I  C  T  O  O  O  T  L  E  R  I  L  O  T  R
N  O  V  T  L  L  L  E  U  T  R  C  X  E  G  A  I  E  P  C
A  R  T  I  C  U  L  A  T  I  O  N  N  E  G  E  H  O  R  L
S  Y  N  O  V  I  A  L  G  T  T  E  T  E  N  D  O  N  O  C
I  C  E  A  R  I  L  G  T  E  G  C  N  V  O  O  L  I  S  M
Y  R  M  R  A  G  A  A  A  E  O  G  A  N  C  V  O  O  E  C
N  R  M  N  R  A  C  C  D  E  T  D  I  P  V  O  M  M  R  N
H  N  G  L  R  C  O  M  V  O  E  C  D  M  M  V  L  I  I  O
O  M  I  R  T  R  A  E  I  C  A  M  N  L  L  O  E  O  E  C
P  E  R  I  O  S  T  E  U  M  E  A  V  E  E  N  C  M  L  H
A  C  M  N  A  S  L  M  E  O  T  E  O  R  R  E  C  E  V  C
```

1. Articulation- _____

2. Bursa- _____

3. Cancellous- _____

4. Cartilage- _____

5. Collagen- _____

6. Compact- _____

7. Degenerative- _____

8. Extremities- _____

9. Ligament- _____

10. Marrow- _____

11. Orthopedic-_____

12. Periosteum-_____

13. Resorption-_____

14. Synovial-_____

15. Tendon-_____

Just the Facts

1. Bone tissue is composed of inorganic ◯ _ _ _ _, blood vessels, nerves, and

   _ _ _ _ _ _ _ _ _.

2. The skeletal system consists of two major groups called the ◯ _ _ _ _ skeleton and the

   _ _ _ _ _ _ _ ◯ _ _ _ _ _ skeleton.

3. Bones are classified by _ _ _ _ _ as long, short, flat, or irregular.

4. The sinus cavities make the skull lighter and the voice sound _ ◯ _ _ _ _ _ _ _.

5. The _ _ ◯ _ _ _ _ _ _ _ _ _ are openings in the cranium that close by the

   second year after birth.

6. Freely movable joints include hinge, _ _ _ ◯ _, and _ _ _ _ _ _ _ _ joints.

7. The adult has 32 teeth after the _ _ _ _ _ _ _ _ _ ◯ or primary teeth are

   replaced.

8. Three disorders of the skeletal system that involve an abnormal curvature of the spine

   include _ _ _ _ _ _ _ _ _, _ _ ◯ _ _ _ _ _, and

   _ _ _ ◯ _ _ _ _ _.

9. Two disorders of the skeletal system that involve the teeth include dental _ _ _ _ ◯ _

   and _ ◯ _ _ _ _ _ _ _ _ _ _ _ _.

10. A common disorder of the skeletal system that is a repetitive stress injury is

    _ _ ◯ _ _ _ _ _ _ _ _ _ _ _ _ _ _ _ _ _ ◯ _.

Use the circled letters to form the answer to this jumble. Clue: What is one of the functions of the skeletal system?

_ _ _ _ _   _ _ _ _ _ _ _ _

Concept Applications

Identifying Skeletal Bones

Use Figure 13-1A and B in the textbook to label the diagrams of the anterior and posterior skeletal system in Figure 13-1A and B.

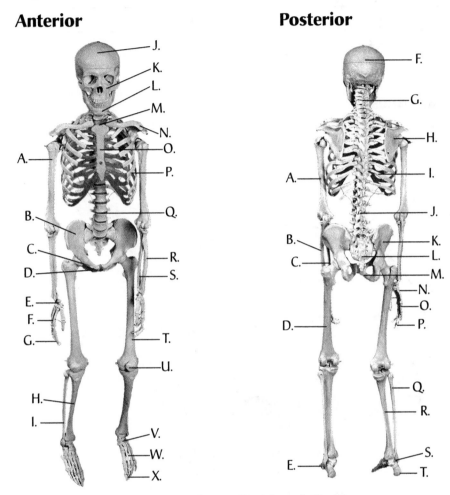

Anterior   **Posterior**

Figure 13-1A and 13-1B

Anterior

A. _____   I. _____   Q. _____

B. _____   J. _____   R. _____

C. _____   K. _____   S. _____

D. _____   L. _____   T. _____

E. _____   M. _____   U. _____

F. _____   N. _____   V. _____

G. _____   O. _____   W. _____

H. _____   P. _____   X. _____

Posterior

A. _____	H. _____	O. _____
B. _____	I. _____	P. _____
C. _____	J. _____	Q. _____
D. _____	K. _____	R. _____
E. _____	L. _____	S. _____
F. _____	M. _____	T. _____
G. _____	N. _____	

Identifying Cranial Bones

Use Figure 13-2 in the textbook to label the diagram of the cranial structures in Figure 13-2.

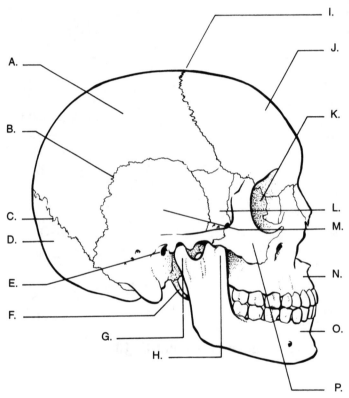

Figure 13-2

A. _____	I. _____
B. _____	J. _____
C. _____	K. _____
D. _____	L. _____
E. _____	M. _____
F. _____	N. _____
G. _____	O. _____
H. _____	P. _____

Identifying Teeth

Use Figure 13-4 in the textbook to label the structures of the tooth in Figure 13-3. Indicate the number of each kind of tooth present in the adult mouth.

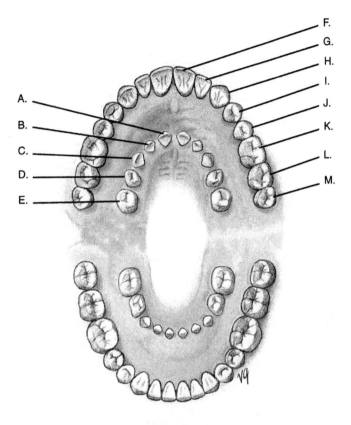

Figure 13-3

A. _____   G. _____

B. _____   H. _____

C. _____   I. _____

D. _____   J. _____

E. _____   K. _____

F. _____   L. _____

                     M. _____

Identifying Structures of the Long Bone

Use Figure 13-8 in the textbook to label the structures of the long bone in Figure 13-4.

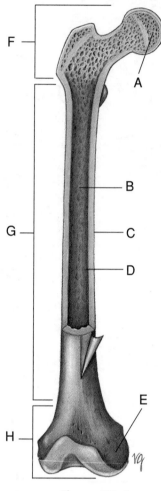

Figure 13-4

A. _____   E. _____
B. _____   F. _____
C. _____   G. _____
D. _____   H. _____

Identifying Disorders of the Skeletal System

Use the textbook to complete the missing information about skeletal system disorders in Table 13-1. Note the etiology (causing factor), signs and symptoms, and treatment and method of prevention (if any).

TABLE 13-1

Disorder	Etiology	Signs and Symptoms	Treatment and Prevention
			Pain medication, bed rest, possible surgical correction
		Abnormal lateral curvature of spine	
	Gout, trauma, infection; may be unknown		
		Inflammation of tissues around teeth; bleeding and tender gums	
		Numbness, tingling, burning sensation in hand	
	Weakening of bones especially in women after menopause		
	Congenital	May cause paralysis and nervous system disorders due to pressure on spinal nerves	

Applying Your Knowledge

1. A group of disorders (usually of unknown cause) that result in stiffness of the joints is collectively called _____.

2. Pressure from repetitive movements of the wrist may lead to a condition called _____ _____. The symptoms of this condition may include _____ and _____.

3. _____ is a condition in which the thoracic spine curves abnormally, whereas _____ is a condition in which the lumbar spine is malformed. Of these two conditions, the one that may cause lower back pain is _____.

4. The condition resulting when bones move out of their normal location but does not include a fracture is called _____.

5. Affecting 90% of adults, the condition that causes most tooth loss in adults is called _____.

Investigations

Cast Application

Plaster casts are applied to the body to immobilize, support, and protest an injured area during healing. They also may be used to prevent or correct bone deformities. Casts are fitted or molded above, around, and below the affected area to provide traction. The material used for casting is usually plaster of Paris or calcium sulfate diphosphate. To make this material, gypsum is reduced to powder by removing the water. The powder can be placed in gauze for easy application. When water is added to the gauze, the plaster hardens and dries in any form.

The bandages for casting are made in varied widths and have "setting" speeds ranging from 2 to 18 minutes to become solid. After being set into a solid form, the process of drying completely takes approximately 10 to 15 minutes longer. The strength of the cast and drying time are determined by the number of layers of gauze applied. Usually five to seven layers are used. Formation of crystals of plaster produces heat during the drying process. A newly set cast is called "green."

The person wearing a cast should be instructed in its proper care to ensure good results from the application. Proper care includes skin care, elevation, isometric exercises, and observation. The area of exposed skin should be washed and dried regularly. Application of lotion on the exposed area will help prevent excess drying of the skin. Massaging the exposed skin will increase circulation and promote comfort. The skin should be inspected regularly to detect any injury such as bruising or damaged skin. A mirror may be used for this purpose if the area is difficult to see.

The skin area under the edge of the cast should be wiped regularly with a washcloth soaked in rubbing alcohol and wrapped around a finger to reduce the sensation of itching. This area under the cast should not be scratched, and foreign objects should not be inserted into the cast. Broken skin under the cast may become infected.

Whenever possible, the area of casting should be elevated to reduce swelling. If a pillow is used to elevate the area, the cast should be secured with a towel pinned to the pillow to prevent accidental slipping. Correct body alignment should be considered at all times to promote comfort and prevent problems resulting from impaired circulation.

Isometric exercises may be used during the time the cast is worn to prevent loss of muscle strength. During exercise, the joint or broken bone should not be moved.

The following are observations that may indicate that a problem has occurred with the casted area. When these conditions occur, the person should be instructed to seek medical attention.

Impaired pulse in the body on the distal end of the cast
Reduced capillary refill (speed of blood return to toe or fingernails)
Musty smell
Increase in body temperature
A warm or hot spot on the skin around the casting area
Tingling sensation
Numbness
Swelling
Coldness of skin
Pale or cyanotic (bluish) skin
Paralysis
Draining from casting area
Nausea, vomiting, abdominal pain, and distention may indicate cast syndrome with a full body cast.

Disposable gloves may be worn, if preferred, because the plaster may stick to the hands of the person applying the cast. Read all directions before beginning the activity. Laboratory activities should be performed only under the supervison of a qualified professional. To prevent accidental injury, casting is practiced on a mannequin.

Equipment and Supplies

alcohol
bucket of warm water
gloves
knife
mannequin
plastic wrap
soap
stockinette

Directions

1. The skin around the area of cast application is prepared by cleaning with soap and water. Alcohol may be used to dry the skin thoroughly. Some physicians also apply talcum powders to prepare the skin.

2. Place a soft knit material or stockinette over the area to be casted.

3. Sheet wadding or padding may be applied over the stockinette. The sheet wadding and stockinette are applied smoothly to prevent skin breakdown from wrinkling. Liquid adhesive may also be used.

4. Line two buckets and the table surface to be used with plastic. The plaster material will bind permanently to many surfaces. Plaster waste is never disposed of in sinks because it will solidity in the piping.

5. Place lukewarm water in the buckets. The temperature of the water determines how fast the plaster sets. Warmer water speeds the setting time and also produces more heat during drying.

6. Grasp the plaster roll by placing your thumb in the middle of the roll.

7. Submerse the roll of plaster vertically (on end) into the water.

8. When bubbles stop rising from the rolls grasp both ends of the bandage to prevent unraveling and remove it from the water.

9. Squeeze the bandage slightly to remove water by forming a bulge in the center of the roll. Do not twist or wring the bandage. Plaster bandages are aplied when still soppy wet.

10. The part to be casted must be kept in the correct alignment, or position, throughout the procedure. After the procedure the area may be radiographed to confirm correct alignment.

11. The plaster bandage is wrapped around the area from the most distal end toward the heart. Each roll is applied so that it covers half of the width of the previous roll. Bandages are applied directly over the stockinette fitting closely, but not tightly enough to hinder circulation in the area. Bandages may be soaked two at a time for quicker application. If bandages soak in the water too long, some of the plaster material may be lost.

12. Smooth the edges and surface of the cast by rubbing the cast with an open hand in a continuous motion during application.

13. Trim the plaster with a knife as necessary to smooth edges or provide windows for circulation and observation of tissues.

14. Casts may be split on both sides (bivalve) to relieve pressure from swelling if needed. Remove excess plaster from the skin with a solution of vinegar and water on a damp sponge.

15. Position the cast in an elevated position after the cast has cooled. During drying, the cast should be exposed to the air to allow the release of the heat produced. The wet cast should not be handled roughly to avoid indentation from fingers that might cause pressure sores.

16. Observe the cast for evidence of drying. The characteristics in Box 13-1 may be used to determine if a cast has dried.

Box 13-1

Wet Cast	Dry Cast
musty smell	odorless
dull sound when tapped	hollow sound when tapped
gray and lusterless	white and shiny
cool to touch	room temperature

Drawing Conclusions

1. What might the presence of numbness, tingling, or paralysis in a limb with a cast indicate?

_____

_____

_____

2. What might the presence of pale or cyanotic skin indicate?

_____

_____

_____

3. What might draining from the casting area indicate?

_____

_____

_____

4. Why is a stockinette used for skin preparation?

_____

_____

_____

Critical Thinking

Rheumatoid Conditions

Rheumatoid refers to the tissues around the joints. Rheumatoid conditions are chronic, disabling, and usually incurable. They include rheumatoid arthritis, systemic lupus erythematosus, progressive systemic sclerosis, Lyme disease, and myositis, as well as many types of arthritis. More than 60 million Americans have a form of rheumatic disease.

Edema resulting from rheumatoid conditions may be managed with aspirin or aspirin-like NSAIDs (nonsteroidal antiinflammatory drugs). Pain relievers and exercise programs help the person retain use of the affected joints. In some cases, corticosteroids may be administered and surgery may be used to correct resulting deformities. In some specific cases, antimalarial drugs, gold salts, penicillamine, sulfasalazine, and immunosuppressive agents may be used to control symptoms. Diet also may have a positive effect. People with rheumatoid conditions have been the victims of many types of quackery.

More than 60 million Americans have a form of rheumatic disease.

Examining the Evidence

1. Why do you think that people with rheumatoid conditions would be candidates for a quackery cure or treatment?

   _____

   _____

   _____

2. Some victims of the AIDS virus develop arthritis. What do you think might be the relation of this condition with the rheumatoid conditions?

   _____

   _____

   _____

3. Management of rheumatoid conditions is expensive due to the necessary medications and treatments. What are two methods by which the costs may be reduced?

   _____

   _____

   _____

14 Muscular System

Vapid Vocabulary

Before reading the chapter, challenge your knowledge of words used in the chapter by completing the crossword puzzle of glossary terms.

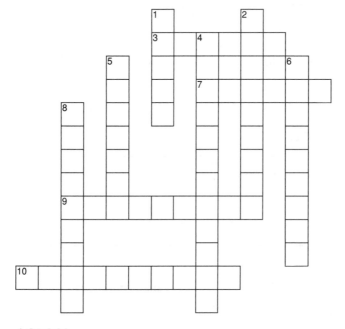

ACROSS

3 An involuntary action in response to a stimulus
7 Removal and examination of living tissue
9 Sitting habitually, inactive habits
10 Something that sticks out from its surroundings

DOWN

1 Depression between thigh and trunk, inguinal region
2 Distortion of any part or disfigurement of the body
4 Quivering or spontaneous contraction of individual muscle fibers
5 Weak, soft
6 Lack of sameness on both sides of the body in size, shape, and relative position
8 Decrease in symptoms of a disease

Key Search

Find the Key Terms from the chapter in the word search puzzle below. Define each of the terms in the space provided.

```
A  C  P  R  T  S  M  P  S  O  E  E  N  P  T  R  O  T  U  A
Y  E  O  I  E  Y  H  T  A  R  T  O  H  S  Y  O  I  T  N  I
C  C  C  N  A  V  I  R  U  P  I  H  I  Y  H  P  O  R  T  A
A  A  H  L  T  M  O  T  P  T  S  N  A  T  E  O  O  L  A  T
E  O  G  H  U  R  C  M  O  C  O  P  I  O  E  O  T  I  A  U
I  I  A  L  C  A  A  M  E  G  O  E  S  P  O  I  O  O  A  P
A  O  U  N  R  H  F  C  A  M  N  U  O  I  A  O  N  S  P  E
M  S  H  T  N  O  A  T  T  L  I  A  O  H  A  I  U  A  T  P
N  R  N  H  E  K  N  P  C  I  A  R  S  K  C  C  I  I  P  I
P  O  M  G  C  A  A  E  P  E  O  T  P  A  O  P  A  P  E  T
C  A  N  R  P  E  U  N  E  I  C  N  E  T  N  U  R  V  H  H
R  A  R  P  O  L  E  C  C  K  N  C  D  L  S  O  I  O  A  G
R  S  S  A  R  C  O  M  E  R  E  O  Y  A  E  S  T  S  O  O
L  M  N  T  L  C  H  U  A  U  S  M  S  M  C  K  U  E  G  A
H  O  O  S  A  Y  O  A  C  F  K  C  T  E  S  N  S  K  H  T
M  G  U  T  N  O  S  N  Y  C  T  L  R  O  O  P  S  T  L  V
C  O  L  N  L  T  S  I  O  A  P  A  O  T  P  I  A  M  A  P
A  N  N  E  U  M  I  R  S  U  L  E  P  E  R  U  T  S  O  P
A  L  O  R  G  L  E  O  M  O  I  A  H  T  E  M  M  N  E  P
O  I  O  U  C  L  O  O  V  H  T  R  Y  S  U  N  C  U  P  P
```

1. Antagonist- _____

2. Atrophy- _____

3. Contraction- _____

4. Contracture- _____

5. Dystrophy-_____

6. Myalgia-_____

7. Paralysis- _____

8. Posture- _____

9. Prime mover-_____

10. Range of motion-_____

11. Sarcomere-_____

12. Skeletal-_____

13. Stimulus-_____

14. Tonus-_____

15. Visceral-_____

Just the Facts

1. Muscle contraction is the Ⓞ _ _ _ _ _ _ _ of muscles when stimulated.

2. _ _ _ _ Ⓞ is the muscle's ability to maintain slight, continuous contraction.

3. Skeletal muscle tissue looks striated, or Ⓞ _ _ _ _ _, under the microscope.

4. The three parts of the skeletal muscle are the _ _ _ _ _ _ _,
   _ _ _ _ _ _ _ _ _ _, and Ⓞ _ _ _ _ _ _.

5. _ _ _ _ Ⓞ _ _ _ muscle lines various hollow organs, makes up the walls of blood
   vessels, and is found in the tubes of the digestive system.

6. Cardiac muscle is found only in the heart and is Ⓞ _ _ _ _ _ _ _ _ _ _ _
   striated.

7. _ Ⓞ _ _ _ _ _ _ _ _ _ is a condition in which muscles remain contracted as
   a joint loses flexibility and ligaments and tendons shorten.

8. Two muscular system disorders that are caused by bacteria are _ _ Ⓞ _ _ _ _ _
   and _ _ _ _ _ _ _.

9. A muscular system disorder that includes a genetic cause in one form is
   _ _ _ Ⓞ _ _ _ _ _ _ _ _ _ _ _ _ _ Ⓞ _.

10. When choosing a sports club, some factors that should be considered include the
    credentials of the _ _ _ _ _, _ _ _ _ _ of the facility,
    _ _ _ _ _ _ Ⓞ _ _ _ _, and Ⓞ _ _ _ _ _ _ _ terms.

Use the circled letters to form the answer to this jumble. Clue: What is a new trend in sports
medicine that studies the body in motion?

_ _ _ _ _ _ _ _ _ _ _ _

Concept Applications

Identifying Anterior Muscles

Use Figure 14-1A in the textbook to label the diagram of the anterior muscles in Figure 14-1. The human body has more than 200 bones.

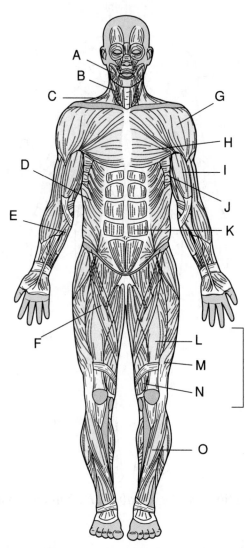

Figure 14-1 Courtesy of Sorrentino: *Mosby's Textbook for Nursing Assistants,* ed 5, Hanover, 2000, Mosby Lifeline.

A. _____   F. _____   K. _____

B. _____   G. _____   L. _____

C. _____   H. _____   M. _____

D. _____   I. _____   N. _____

E. _____   J. _____   O. _____

Identifying Posterior Muscles

Use Figure 14-1B in the textbook to label the diagram of the posterior muscles in Figure 14-2.

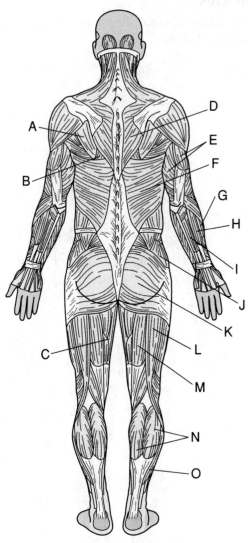

Figure 14–2 Courtesy of Sorrentino: *Mosby's Textbook for Nursing Assistants,* ed 5, Hanover, 2000, Mosby Lifeline.

A. _____   F. _____   K. _____

B. _____   G. _____   L. _____

C. _____   H. _____   M. _____

D. _____   I. _____   N. _____

E. _____   J. _____   O. _____

Identifying Muscle Tissue Types

Use Figures 14-2, 14-6, and 14-7 in the textbook to label the diagrams of muscle tissue type in Figure 14-3A to C in the spaces provided in Table 14-1. Indicate whether each of the muscle types is controlled by voluntary or involuntary action.

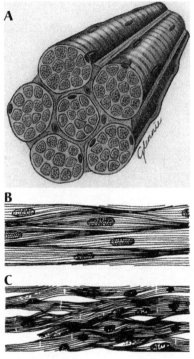

Figure 14-3

TABLE 14-1

Tissue Type	Type of Action (Voluntary or Involuntary)
A. _____	_____
B. _____	_____
C. _____	_____

Identifying Disorders of the Muscular System

Use the textbook to complete the missing information about muscular system disorders in Table 14-2. Note the etiology (causing factor), signs and symptoms, and treatment and method of prevention (if any).

TABLE 14-2

Disorder	Etiology	Signs and Symptoms	Treatment and Prevention
	Genetic		
			Bracing, surgical procedure to restore proper positioning and medication
		Joint loses flexibility, tendons may shorten	
			Treatment includes preventing complications, may be prevented with vaccination
	Viral infection		
	Clostridium bacteria		
	Cause unknown, considered to be autoimmune		

Applying Your Knowledge

1. Loss of flexibility in a joint resulting in a shortening of the tendons and ligaments is called a

    _____ and may be caused by _____.

2. Painless, gradual atrophy of the muscles may be caused by a genetic condition called

    _____ _____.

3. Often occurring in the groin area, the condition called a _____ may be treated with surgery.

4. Paralysis caused by _____ may be prevented by a vaccination.

5. Caused by the *Clostridium* bacteria, _____ may lead to the death of muscle tissue.

Investigations

Observing Muscle Tissue

Read all directions before beginning the activity. Laboratory activities should be performed only under the supervision of a qualified professional. Care must be taken when handling chemicals and glassware. Gloves are worn when handling raw meat products.

Equipment and Supplies

disposable gloves
dissecting needle
eyedropper
forceps
methylene blue stain
microscope
microscope slides and cover slips
prepared slide of muscle tissue types
raw pork chop or beef

Directions

1. Examine a prepared slide of each of the three muscle types under low and high power.

2. Draw each of the three muscle types as observed under high power in the spaces provided in Figure 14-4. Label the nucleus, cytoplasm, cell membrane, and striations that can be identified.

3. In a drop of water on a clean slide, tease apart a small piece of raw meat. Separate the fibers with a dissecting needle.

4. Transfer a few strands of the meat fiber to a slide that has been prepared with a dry film of dilute methylene blue stain.

5. Add a drop of water and cover slip to the slide. Wrap the slide and cover slip in paper toweling and gently press with the thumb or a pencil eraser to spread the fibers.

6. Observe the slide under low and then high power. Draw the specimen as observed under high power in the space provided in Figure 14-5.

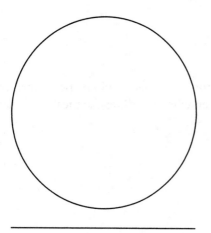

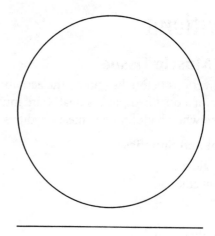

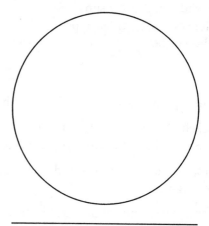

Figure 14-4

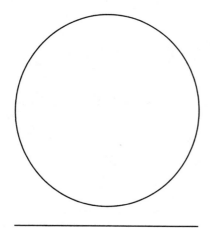

Figure 14-5

Drawing Conclusions

1. Which of the prepared muscle slides looks most like the slide that you made?

_____

_____

_____

2. Which of the prepared muscle tissue slides is the most easily identified by microscopic examination? Explain why this is so.

_____

_____

_____

3. Based on the observation of the slide you prepared, what do you think happens to the muscle tissue in a muscle tear injury?

_____

_____

_____

Observing Muscle Movement

Read all directions before beginning the activity. Laboratory activities should be performed only under the supervision of a qualified professional. Care must be taken when handling chemicals and glassware. Gloves are worn when handling raw meat products.

Equipment and Supplies

raw chicken wing   forceps
disposable gloves   paper towels
dissecting tray   scissors

Directions

1. Rinse a whole raw chicken wing under running water. Dry it with paper towels and place it in a dissecting tray.

2. Pull the skin away from the muscle with forceps and cut the skin the length of the wing. Care should be taken to avoid cutting the underlying muscle tissue. Observe the thin connective tissue (mesentery) between the skin and muscle tissues.

3. With a probe, separate the skin from the muscle. If the skin over the joints is difficult to remove, a scalpel may be used in this area. It is not necessary to remove the skin from the wing tip.

4. Rinse and dry the chicken wing after removing the skin. Observe and diagram the chicken wing in the space provided in Figure 14-6.

5. Observe the tendons at the end of the muscles. Notice the shape of the muscles.

6. Grasp the wing at the shoulder and tip. Pull the wing to extend the length and bend it back to its original shape. Observe how the muscles contract during movement. Identify the muscles that work in pairs.

7. Observe the largest muscle of the wing to determine its origin and insertion.

8. Draw the chicken wing as it appears after removal of the skin. Label the muscle origin, insertion, body, tendons, and bones in Figure 14-7. Use arrows to indicate the direction of the antagonistic muscles in the diagram.

9. Dispose of the chicken wing and gloves in the appropriate container. Clean laboratory equipment and replace it to the designated area as instructed.

10. Wash your hands thoroughly with soap and water.

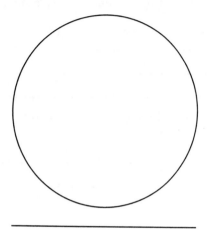

Figure 14-6

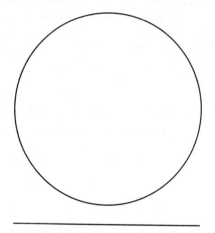

Figure 14-7

Drawing Conclusions

1. Use Figure 14-4 in the textbook to name two antagonistic, or opposing, muscles in the human body.

   _____

   _____

   _____

2. Why are disposable gloves worn when handling raw meat?

   _____

   _____

   _____

Demonstrating Reflex Actions

Muscles contract when they are stimulated, manipulated, or pulled by gravity. They also contract when the tendons attaching the muscles are stretched. This activity provides methods of assessing the function of the tendon reflexes. Read all directions before beginning the activity. Laboratory activities should be performed only under the supervision of a qualified professional.

Equipment and Supplies

percussion hammer

Directions

1. Arm reflexes that can be demonstrated include the biceps, triceps, and brachioradialis reflexes. To assess these reflexes, place your thumb over the tendon to hold the limb being observed.

2. Strike your thumb with a percussion hammer so that the blow is transmitted to the tendon. The percussion hammer is held between the thumb and index finger during assessment. Reflexes of both sides of the body should be tested and compared for equality. Table 14-3 indicates the location struck by the percussion hammer and the response expected for these reflexes.

3. Assess the lower limb in a similar manner. The table below provides information about the lower limb reflexes and expected responses.

TABLE 14-3

Disorder	Location of Thumb	Expected Response
Biceps	The arm is flexed at the elbow with the examiner's thumb over the biceps tendon in the antecubital area (Fig. 14-8A).	Flexion of the arm at the elbow
Triceps	The arm is flexed at the elbow with the examiner's thumb over the triceps tendon on the outer aspect of the arm (Fig. 14-8B).	Straightening or extension of the arm
Brachioradialis	Examiner's thumb supports extended arm in a relaxed position while the styloid process (bony prominence on wrist) is struck with hammer (Fig. 14-8C).	Flexion of the arm at the elbow
Patellar	With legs dangling free over side of chair or bed, tap directly below or inferior to the patella (Fig. 14-8D).	Extension of the leg
Achilles tendon	Foot is held in slight dorsiflexed position (Fig. 14-8E).	Plantar flexion of the foot
Plantar	Use a key, pin, or the end of the reflex hammer to press a line from the lateral border of the sole starting at the heel and continuing up to and across the ball of the foot (Fig. 14-8F).	Flexion of all of the toes

4. Record the results of the activity in Table 14-4. Use a "+" sign to indicate a reaction and a "−" to indicate no response

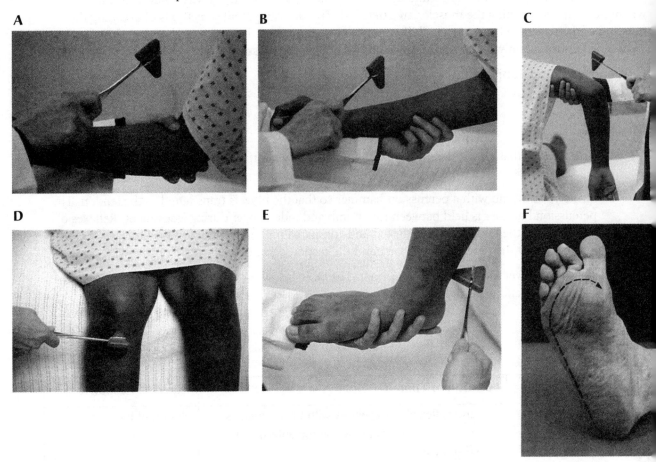

Figure 14-8 Courtesy of Seidel: *Mosby's Guide to Physical Examination,* ed 5, St. Louis, 2003, Mosby.

TABLE 14–4

Reflex	Right Side Response	Left Side Response
Biceps	_____	_____
Triceps	_____	_____
Brachioradialis	_____	_____
Patellar	_____	_____
Achilles tendon	_____	_____
Plantar	_____	_____

Drawing Conclusions

1. Which of the reflexes tested showed a positive response?

_____

_____

_____

2. Which of the reflexes showed a negative response? Hypothesize why these responses were absent.

_____

_____

_____

3. List three factors that might influence the results of this activity.

_____

_____

_____

Critical Thinking

Muscles of the Face and Neck

Study the diagram of the muscles of the head and face in Figure 14-9. In the space provided in Table 14-5, list the muscles that you think may be involved in the actions listed.

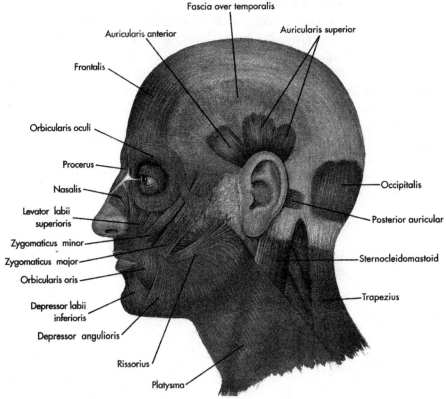

Figure 14-9 Courtesy of Seidel: *Mosby's Guide to Physical Examination,* ed 5, St. Louis, 2003, Mosby.

TABLE 14-5

Action	Muscles Involved in the Action
1. Smile	
2. Blink	
3. Tension headache	
4. Sneeze	
5. Moving Ear	
6. Chewing	
7. Yawning	

Weight Training

Body-building by using weights or weight training became popular with increased interest in health and fitness. It is estimated that more than 7 million Americans exercise regularly with weights. Equipment and exercise routines have been developed to improve the strength and muscle tone in all areas of the body. After only 6 weeks of training, the benefits of weight training can be seen in the development of firmer and stronger muscles.

A high-protein diet promotes muscle mass.

Lifting weights causes the proteins that form muscle tissue to pull apart. The muscle tissue is broken down and then replaced with new tissue. The new tissue has bigger and stronger fibers than those that were destroyed. The body requires about 48 hours to regenerate the proteins of muscle tissues. For that reason, it is not a good idea to exercise the same muscle groups every day.

Weight training is an anaerobic exercise, which means it does not consume oxygen. It uses energy that is stored in the muscles. Some exercise equipment is designed for continuous use to increase cardio-vascular or aerobic benefit from lifting weights. However, combining aerobic movement and stretching with lifting weights provides an all-around fitness program.

Weights may be used in either free form or as part of a machine. Free weights, barbells, and dumb-bells are not as expensive as the machinery designed for weight training. The correct equipment should be selected for the results desired.

Precautions such as the use of correct body mechanics and stretching exercises must be taken to prevent injury during use of all types of weights. All weight-training programs should begin slowly to prevent torn or damaged muscles and tendons.

Examining the Evidence

1. Why is the addition of stretching exercises and aerobic activity to weight training a complete program of fitness?

   _____

   _____

   _____

2. If a person desires to lift weights every day, how could a program be designed to prevent muscle injury?

   _____

   _____

   _____

3. What precautions are used to prevent muscle tears when lifting weights?

   _____

   _____

   _____

15 *Digestive System*

Vapid Vocabulary

Before reading the chapter, challenge your knowledge of words used in the chapter by completing the crossword puzzle of glossary terms.

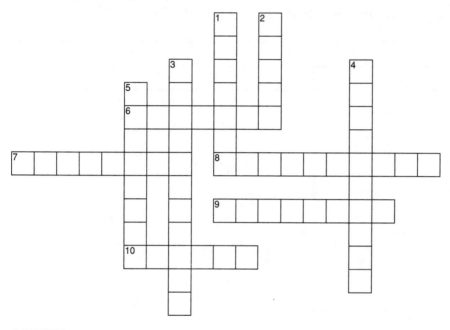

ACROSS

6 Localized collection of pus in a cavity, formed by destruction of tissue
7 Indigestible material such as fibers in diet
8 Situated at right angles, placed crosswise
9 Apparatus to bathe the perineal area with continuous flow of fluid
10 A protein that accelerates specific chemical reaction

DOWN

1 Organic material that gives color in the body
2 Excrement discharged from intestines
3 Milk or other liquids that have been heated to a moderate temperature for a definite time to kill pathogenic bacteria
4 Hurled or propelled forward
5 Agent that acts to promote evacuation of the bowel; cathartic

Key Search

Find the Key Terms from the chapter in the word search puzzle below. Define each of the terms in the space provided.

```
Y M O T C E T S Y C E L O H C D N N U I
S U A E H N Y P O C S O D N E E O O S M
T I U C Y E E M N E L N I D C G I I I G
B L S M M M U E L L T I L I U L T T S L
N U L L E A L L L I D B D T N U A S E S
N S U F A U M C D B O N I C N T C E M I
N T F U T T M I M Y U T I C T I I G E G
O C T A P L S O B A N U Y E V T T N S A
N O L L N H L I J U B O S N I I S I O D
G F P Y F E E Y R I L O U N L O A D G V
E D D O N O A F C E I I T O L N M N B N
D E F E C A T I O N P U M N U H G F U M
O T E T S T D D T N E I O I S B D C I D
S P H I N C T E R O E T T I A S U I O I
L N U O T G T B T O T E T S N O B Y I C
T O O L D C E T O M F I O M E E L U T D
I O S V V U N L S L D O C G C T H U P M
A I S A T C A L A L U C O Y Y B M F C A
E S U N N C O B N T A S U Y L N U V L Y
B S O N P I S Y N G M E L S C A S T A E
```

1. Alactasia- _____

2. Bile- _____

3. Bolus- _____

4. Bulimia-_____

5. Cholecystectomy- _____

6. Chyme- _____

7. Defecation- _____

8. Deglutition-_____

9. Emesis- _____

10. Endoscopy- _____

11. Enema- _____

12. Flatulence-_____

13. Ingestion- _____

14. Jaundice- _____

15. Mastication-_____

16. Peristalsis- _____

17. Sphincter- _____

18. Villus- _____

Just the Facts

1. The main function of the digestive system is to _ _ _ ◯ _ _ _ _ _ food to a form that can be used by ◯ _ _ _ _ _ _ _ _ _.

2. Three _ _ ◯ _ _ _ _ _ glands secrete an enzyme (amylase) that begins the chemical portion of the digestive process in the _ ◯ _ _ _.

3. In the stomach, the food _ _ _ ◯ _ mixes with hydrochloric acid and the enzymes pepsin and gastrin to become _ _ _ _ _.

4. Most absorption of digestive products occurs in the _ _ _ _ _ _ _ ◯ _ _ _ _ _ _ _.

5. Most of the water from ingested food is absorbed back into the blood through the walls of the _ ◯ _ _ _ _ _ _ _ _ _ _ _ _ _ _,

6. The digestive system has three accessory organs, which that aid the process of food breakdown. They are the _ _ ◯ _ _ _ _ _ _, _ _ _ _ _ _ _ _ _ _ _ _ _, and _ ◯ _ _ _.

7. The liver has many important functions including storage of _ _ _ _ _ _ _ and _ _ _ _ _ ◯ _ _, break down of _ _ _ ◯ _ _, and reprocessing of _ _ _ ◯ _ _ _ _ _ _ _ _ _ _.

8. Two digestive system disorders that involve problems with elimination are ◯ _ _ _ _ _ _ _ and _ _ _ _ _ _ _ _ _ _ _ _.

9. Two digestive system disorders that have a genetic cause are _ _ _ _ ◯ _ _ _ _ _ _ _ _ _ _ _ and _ _ _◯ _ _ _ _.

10. Two digestive system disorders that are caused by a virus are _ $\bigcirc$ _ _ _ _ _ _ _
and the $\bigcirc$ _ _ _ _ _.

Use the circled letters to form the answer to this jumble. Clue: What are two of the most common eating disorders called?

_ _ _ _ _ _ _ _   _ _ _ _ _ _ _ _ _ _ _ _

Concept Applications

Identifying Structures and Functions of the Digestive System

Use Figure 15-1 in the textbook to label the diagram of the digestive system in Figure 15-1. In the spaces provided in Table 15-1, describe the function of each part.

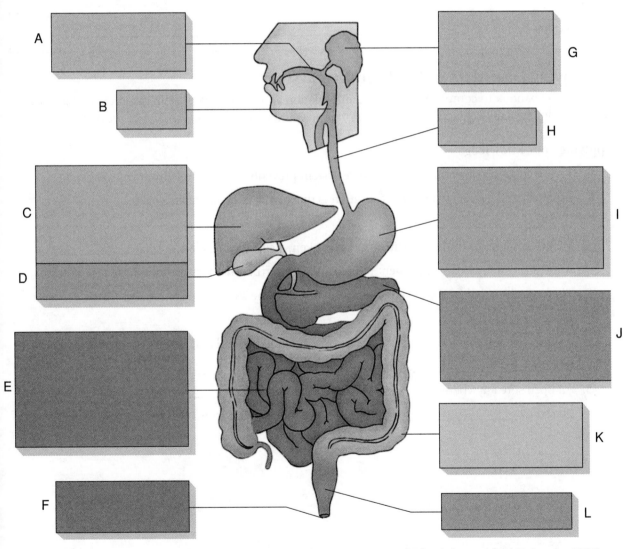

Figure 15-1 Courtesy of Thibodeau GA, Patton KT: *Anatomy and Physiology*, ed 4, St. Louis, 1999, Mosby.

TABLE 15-1

Organ	Function
1. Mouth	
2. Esophagus	
3. Stomach	
4. Small intestine	
5. Pharnyx	
6. Salivary glands	
7. Large intestine	
8. Rectum	
9. Anus	
10. Gallbladder	
11. Liver	
12. Pancreas	

Identifying Disorders of the Digestive System

Use the textbook to complete the missing information about digestive system disorders in Table 15-2. Note the etiology (causing factor), signs and symptoms, and treatment and method of prevention (if any).

Applying Your Knowledge

1. A very common disorder of the digestive system prevents many people from enjoying milk products such as ice cream. This condition is due to a lack of an enzyme called

   _____.

2. When radiographs of the intestinal tract are taken, a substance called _____ is sometimes swallowed by the client to help show the structures as it passes through the tract.

3. The procedure that may be used to view the inside of the stomach or to remove gastric contents is called _____.

4. A viral infection that may result from eating contaminated food and that causes jaundice affects the _____. This condition is called _____.

5. An open sore anywhere along the digestive tract is called an _____ and may be caused by _____ that eats the lining of the stomach.

TABLE 15-2

Disorder	Etiology	Signs and Symptoms	Treatment and Prevention
	Virus, transmitted in food or water or in body secretions		
	Salmonella and other bacteria		
			Emotion and stress may trigger symptoms; diet changes, medication, surgery
	Bacteria or stress		
		Flatulence, cramps, diarrhea when dairy products are ingested	
		Jaundice, skin lesions, demineralization of bones, enlargement of the liver, anemia, bleeding disorders	
			Surgical removal of the appendix

Investigations

Dissection of a Perch

Read all of the directions before beginning this activity. Disposable gloves are worn while handling specimens if prepared or stored in caustic fluids. Directions are for dissection of preserved perch. Pigeons, fetal pigs, and frogs may be used as well.

Equipment and Supplies

disposable gloves
preserved specimen (perch)
dissecting tray
forceps
dissection scissors

Directions

1. Place the specimen for dissection on a dissecting tray.

2. Examine the teeth of the specimen, taking care not to be cut by the sharp edges. Observe the mouth cavity.

3. Using forceps and a pair of scissors, open the abdominal cavity of the specimen carefully to avoid cutting the organs.

4. Observe the membrane surrounding the abdominal organs. Carefully loosen this membrane and move it to the side.

5. Locate the esophagus of the perch. The esophagus leads directly into the saclike stomach pouch. Observe the shape and size of the stomach.

6. The stomach leads into the intestine. The waste of the perch leaves the body through the rectum. Trace the intestine to the rectum.

7. Locate and observe the liver of the perch. Observe that the gallbladder is attached to the liver.

8. Observe that the stomach is attached to the intestine by a small tube or duct.

9. Label the following parts of the digestive system of the perch on the diagram in Figure 15-2.

mouth	stomach
intestine	anus
teeth	liver
gallbladder	esophagus

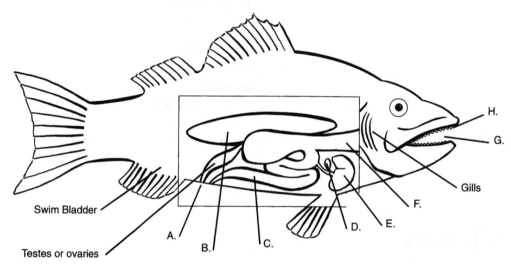

Figure 15-2

A.	_____	E.	_____
B.	_____	F.	_____
C.	_____	G.	_____
D.	_____	H.	_____

Drawing Conclusions

1. The small fish and aquatic organisms eaten by the perch are swallowed whole. What purpose do the teeth and mouth serve?

_____

_____

_____

2. The stomach of the perch is much larger than its liver. In humans, the liver is larger than the stomach. How would you explain this difference?

_____

_____

_____

3. Based on your observations of the perch's digestive system, hypothesize whether it would get more nutrition from eating frequently or less often.

_____

_____

_____

Critical Thinking

Understanding Eating Disorders

Some authorities believe that the origin of eating disorders is related to a victim's need to have control of some feature of his/her life such as appearance. By exerting control over the body by losing weight despite hunger and signs of physical damage, the victim of the disorder feels a sense of power. Often victims believe they are fat even when they are extremely thin. The theory continues that weight loss gives the victim a sense of identify or feeling of being competent because he/she is able to lose weight.

Authorities estimate that 2% to 8% of adolescent and college-age women in the United States suffer from bulimia.

Examining Evidence

1. When eating disorders, such as anorexia nervosa and bulimia, result in obvious physical changes, such as hair loss and tooth damage, why do you think these changes do not stop the victim from purging or self-starvation?

_____

_____

_____

2. According to the American Anorexia/Bulimia Association, approximately 1% of all teenagers suffer from anorexia. Men represent 5% to 10% of all eating disorders. Of college-age women, 5% to 20% are reportedly bulimic. These numbers are increasing. Hypothesize at least one reason for the increase in frequency of this disorder.

_____

_____

_____

3. Some of the signs of eating disorders include rapid weight gain or loss, preoccupation with calories, denial or defensive behavior when confronted with eating habits, unexplained vomiting, sores at the corners of the mouth, and continuous episodes of overeating without weight gain. If you observed these signs in someone you knew, what would you do?

_____

_____

_____

16 Urinary System

Vapid Vocabulary

Before reading the chapter, challenge your knowledge of words used in the chapter by completing the crossword puzzle of glossary terms.

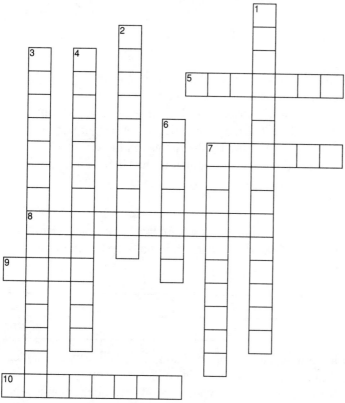

ACROSS

5 Proper care of the mouth, teeth, and other parts of the body for maintenance of health and the prevention of disease

7 Foul, unpleasant

8 Arrangement into proper proportion or relation; qualitative and quantitative makeup of chemical compound

9 White substance found in urine, blood, and lymph; end product of protein digestion

10 Pertaining to a group of interdependent parts or organs

DOWN

1 Movement of materials across cell membrane and epithelial layers requiring energy
2 Passage of liquid through a filter by gravity, pressure, or suction fissure cleft or groove; linear ulcer flaccid weak, soft
3 Weight of a substance compared to an equal volume of another substance (usually water) used as a standard
4 Permitting the passage of certain molecules and not others
6 Quality of being clear, lucid
7 Pertaining to the layer of membrane lining the abdominopelvic walls

Key Search

Find the Key Terms from the chapter in the word search puzzle below. Define each of the terms in the space provided.

```
A S I S Y L A I D R O A I I N C D A A I
I O I N A A T N N I I G L I A G H I A N
R I I A R C R A S R I A I N T L E R N A
U R U R A P R A N A U U O R S U M P I I
N Y I I A O I O N R I R O I U O A G I G
I I T I S I D R A G C R I L L A T S A O
M G U I A I O R N L S I U L R N U I I R
U G O D R U I L A I I A P S T I R A O G
B G L Y C O S U R I A Y I R Y U I N R O
L H I R S S I S E R U I D R Y D A N A D
A N U R I A Y R C R A O I L A I I O D D
O Y O L I A O L I G I G O O A T U L A O
L R L A O N L A A S C P U S O A D R I R
A C I A A O N A A A I Y S A I L I S G Y
R D G I R N O I T I R U T C I M O D A A
R A U I D R D S I I R S O R O A V A S L
I A R G N A L S I S E U T E R I O T L U
U R I N A L Y S I S N R R Y A T A O R I
R G A U U S N L O B E N S R N L R I I I
T P I I I O R I U R I N A T I O N R A I
```

1. Albuminuria-_____

2. Anuria- _____

3. Dialysis-_____

4. Diuresis- _____

5. Dysuria-_____

6. Glycosuria- _____

7. Hematuria- _____

8. Micturition-_____

9. Oliguria- _____

10. Polyuria- _____

11. Pyuria-_____

12. Urinalysis- _____

13. Urination- _____

14. Void- _____

Just the Facts

1. The function of the urinary system includes regulation of the composition of _ _ _ ◯
   ◯ _ _ _ _ _ and removal of _ _ ◯ _ _ _ from the blood.

2. The _ _ ◯ _ _ _ _ is the location of formation of urine and is the functional unit of
   the urinary system.

3. The _ _ _ _ _ _ _, a smooth muscular sac that expands as it fills with urine, can
   hold up to 1 liter.

4. Urine consists of _ _ ◯ _ _ and _ _ _ _ ◯ _ _ _ _ _ _ _ _
   from the breakdown of protein, hormones, electrolytes, pigments, and toxins.

5. Two disorders of the urinary system that are caused by bacteria are
   ◯ _ _ _ _ _ _ _ and _ _ _ _ _ _ _ _ ◯ _ _ _
   _ _ _ _ _ _ _ _ _ _ _.

6. Renal calculi, commonly called kidney stones, are made up of _ _ _ _ _ _ _ _
   and _ _ _ _ ◯ _ _ _ _ _ _ _.

7. Two urinary disorders that involve abnormal excretion or urine are urinary
   _ _ ◯ _ _ _ _ _ _ _ _ _ and urinary _ _ _ _ _ _ _ _ _ _.

8. Two forms of dialysis are _ _ _ _ _ ◯ _ _ _ _ _ _ _ and
   _ _ _ _ _ _ _ _ ◯ _ dialysis.

9. _ ◯ _ _ _ _ _ _ _ _ _ _ _ _ _ _ _ has a success rate of greater
   than 95%.

10. Kidney stones may be removed by _ _ _ Ⓞ _ _ _ or a _ _ _ _ _ _
      _ _ Ⓞ _ treatment called lithotripsy.

Use the circled letters to form the answer to this jumble. Clue: What is a test of the urinary system that shows the density of the urine?

_ _ _ _ _ _ _ _ _ _ _ _ _ _ _ _

Concept Applications

Identifying Structures and Functions of the Urinary System

Use Figure 16-1 in the textbook to label the diagram of the urinary system in Figure 16-1. In the spaces provided in Table 16-1, describe the function of each part.

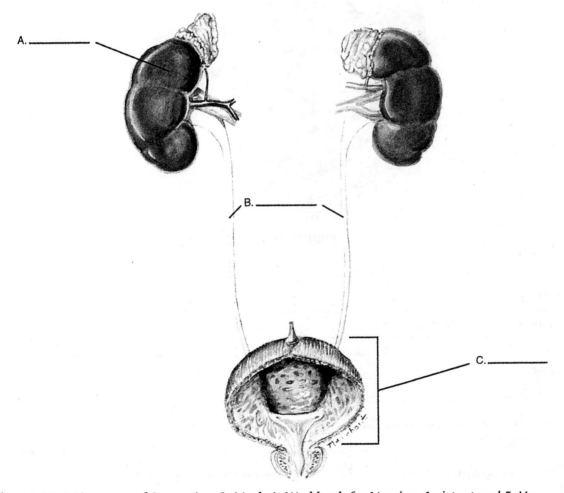

Figure 16-1 Courtesy of Sorrentino S: *Mosby's Workbook for Nursing Assistants,* ed 5, Hanover, 2000, Mosby.

TABLE 16-1

System Part	Main Function
1. Kidney	
2. Ureter	
3. Bladder	

Identifying Structures and Functions of the Kidney

Use Figure 16-3 in the textbook to label the diagram of the cell in Figure 16-2. In the spaces provided in Table 16-2, describe the function of each part.

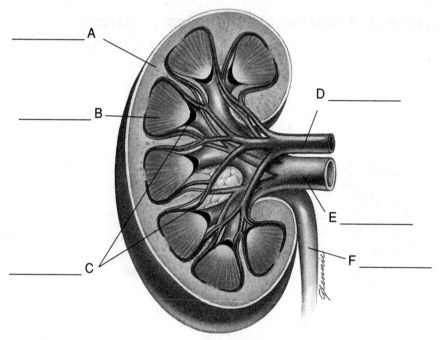

Figure 16-2

TABLE 16-2

Kidney Part	Main Function
1. Cortex	
2. Medulla	
3. Renal pelvis	
4. Renal vein	
5. Renal artery	
6. Ureter	

Identifying Disorders of the Urinary System

Use the textbook to complete the missing information about urinary disorders in Table 16-3. Note the etiology (causing factor), signs and symptoms, and treatment and method of prevention (if any).

TABLE 16-3

Disorder	Etiology	Signs and Symptoms	Treatment and Prevention
		Nausea, vomiting, headache, coma	
		Swollen tissues, locally or systemically	
		Fever; lower back pain; frequent, painful, bloody urination	
	Bacteria	Painful urination, frequency of urination, blood in the urine	
			Lithotripsy or surgical removal might be used
	Bacteria or chemical irritation		
	Lack of muscle control, immobility, neural damage		

Applying Your Knowledge

1. An abnormal amount of fluid accumulation in the tissues of the body is called
   _____. It may be caused by failure of the _____.

2. Another name for a kidney stone is a _____ _____. Its specific cause is _____.

3. Women may suffer a condition called _____ more often than men because the urethra in women is shorter than in men.

4. When the kidneys do not filter the blood, the person may experience nausea, vomiting, headache, and coma. Crystals may form on the skin as the body tries to rid itself of wastes in this condition called _____.

5. The treatment for kidney failure that involves removal of waste products through an artificial kidney is called _____.

Investigations

Urinalysis

Urine composition may be determined by performing a series of simple tests. Read all of the directions before beginning this activity. Disposable gloves are worn when handling body secretions. Laboratory activities should be completed only under the supervision of a qualified professional.

As early as AD 500, urine was studied as an indication of health.

Equipment and Supplies

chemical "dipstick" indicator strip with reference chart
hydrometer or graduated cylinder with urinometer
natural or artificial urine
paper or urine specimen cup
pH paper (or similar acid/base indicator) with reference chart

Directions

1. Collect the appropriate type of urine specimen needed for each test.

2. Observe the clarity of a fresh routine specimen of urine. Record the appearance:

   _____

3. Describe the odor of a fresh routine specimen of urine. Record the smell observed:

   _____

4. Perform a pH test using a fresh routine specimen of urine. Litmus, nitrazine, or hydrion paper may be used as an indicator. Each paper turns varied colors in acidic and basic solutions. Dip the bottom half of a small piece of indicator paper in the specimen. Compare the color of the paper with the chart provided with the paper. Do not touch the paper container with the urine-soaked paper while comparing the colors. Record the value of the pH of the urine:

   _____

5. Perform a specific gravity test using a fresh routine specimen of urine. Pour the urine into a graduated cylinder or hydrometer container to a level 1 inch below the top of the cylinder. Without touching the sides of the cylinder, gently twist and release the urinometer into the urine. Read the results of the specific gravity as soon as the spinning stops. Record the value of the specific gravity:

   _____

6. Use "dipsticks" to determine the presence of any abnormal components of urine including blood, sugar, acetone, and proteins. Follow the manufacturer's instructions for the use of each indicating stick. Record the presence of any abnormal components:

   _____

Drawing Conclusions

1. Use Table 16-2 from your textbook to determine if the observation of clarity made in step two is normal. If the value is outside of the normal range, why might it be different?

   _____

   _____

   _____

2. Use Table 16-2 to determine if the odor noted in step three is normal. If the value is outside of the normal range, why might it be different?

   _____

   _____

   _____

3. In step four, the directions state that care should be taken not to touch the pH paper container with the urine-soaked paper. Why would this be important?

   _____

   _____

   _____

4. Use Table 16-2 to determine if the value obtained for the pH is normal. If the value is not within the normal range, why might it be different?

   _____

   _____

   _____

5. Use Table 16-2 to determine if the value obtained for the specific gravity is normal. If the value is not within the normal range, why might it be different?

   _____

   _____

   _____

6. Use Table 16-2 to determine what the presence of any abnormal components found in the urine specimen might mean and describe the condition.

   _____

   _____

   _____

Critical Thinking

Urinary Changes with Aging

During the aging process, the kidney tissues become scarred and less efficient. Blood vessels carry blood to and from the kidneys at a lower pressure, causing less urine production. Muscle weakness in the pelvic area may lead to urine retention or the inability to empty the bladder completely. In young people, urine is produced throughout the day and concentrated at night. In older individuals, the ability to concentrate urine may be lost, leading to the need to urinate during the night (*nocturia*). The loss of the ability to control urination is called *incontinence*. Incontinence may occur in the elderly due to infection, loss of muscle tone, or an inability to reach the toilet facilities when needed.

Examining the Evidence

1. List three methods that might be used to help an elderly person control a urinary incontinence problem.

   _____

   _____

   _____

2. List two ways in which the problem of nocturia might be lessened.

   _____

   _____

   _____

3. List three physical and/or psychological problems that might result from urinary incontinence or retention.

   _____

   _____

   _____

4. How might you help a person adjust to one of the problems you identified in quesiton three?

   _____

   _____

   _____

Excretion in the Body

In order to complete the chart in Table 16-4, indicate the type of excretion that occurs in each part of the body listed. Make a notation in the "Other Function" column if the body organ listed performs a function other than its urinary system function. Chapter 9 in the textbook provides information about the skin.

TABLE 16-4

| Body Part | Waste Product Removed | | | | | |
	CO_2	Urea	Na^+	Water	Urine	Other Function
Kidneys						
Skin						
Lungs						

Examining the Evidence

1. Sometimes when a person has failure of the kidneys, the skin shows particles of salt. Why would this be true?

   _____

   _____

   _____

2. Sometimes when a person has failure of the kidneys, the skin appears shiny or leatherlike. Why would this be true?

   _____

   _____

   _____

17 *Endocrine System*

Vapid Vocabulary

Before reading the chapter, challenge your knowledge of words used in the chapter by completing the crossword puzzle of glossary terms.

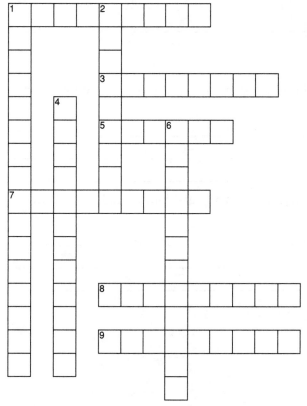

ACROSS

1 Any constructive process by which simple substances are converted by living cells into more complex compounds
3 Condition of drowsiness or indifference
5 Prolonged muscle spasm or contraction
7 Involuntary
8 Process by which glands produce and add chemical substances into the blood, chemical substances
9 Disorder resulting from defective or faulty nutrition

DOWN

1 Counteracting or suppressing inflammation
2 Release of the egg (ovum) from the ovary
4 Cyclic, physiologic discharge through the vagina of blood and mucosal tissues from the nonpregnant uterus
6 Substance suppressing the rate of urine formation

Key Search

Find the Key Terms from the chapter in the word search puzzle below. Define each of the terms in the space provided.

```
Y  E  E  O  G  O  S  G  O  C  L  L  M  S  D  P  O  N  M  P
A  S  N  O  X  S  C  P  O  T  A  O  M  E  L  G  E  S  H  O
I  E  S  I  S  G  H  O  X  N  N  P  P  L  P  M  I  U  O  L
M  E  O  R  R  A  A  O  N  X  A  S  S  O  M  L  P  E  R  Y
E  A  X  L  N  C  M  I  C  Y  Y  D  E  Y  O  E  A  A  M  D
C  M  I  O  B  S  O  G  G  G  C  I  O  B  M  O  H  E  O  I
Y  N  G  M  P  N  I  D  N  A  L  G  A  T  S  O  R  P  N  P
L  A  I  E  E  T  A  A  N  P  H  T  E  M  R  A  G  P  E  S
G  I  P  O  S  C  H  O  O  E  E  P  A  T  M  O  S  H  E  I
R  R  E  E  O  D  Y  A  A  M  A  Y  Y  H  O  M  P  Y  P  A
E  U  P  T  M  I  P  L  L  Y  I  O  L  L  T  O  P  I  P  E
P  Y  R  P  E  O  E  L  G  A  G  P  M  M  O  N  R  A  N  P
Y  L  P  S  A  X  E  Y  P  O  M  S  C  R  R  P  U  S  H  P
H  O  R  S  A  C  T  S  C  M  P  O  Y  T  R  E  B  U  P  M
E  P  G  L  L  L  X  M  A  S  P  Y  S  A  E  N  A  N  O  A
C  G  M  A  T  O  S  A  Y  P  L  E  H  E  A  B  Y  L  T  G
M  A  S  I  M  M  U  N  O  A  S  S  A  Y  Y  S  G  I  O  I
S  A  G  G  A  P  L  C  O  O  N  Y  I  D  M  Y  O  E  R  L
B  E  E  A  Y  Y  O  Y  G  G  M  G  O  P  N  H  Y  M  A  P
O  R  E  N  R  A  C  L  A  N  N  A  Y  E  E  N  M  D  S  G
```

1. Endocrine-_____

2. Exophthalmos- _____

3. Gonadotropin-_____

   4. Hormone- _____

   5. Hyperglycemia- _____

   6. Hypoglycemia- _____

   7. Immunoassay- _____

   8. Polydipsia- _____

   9. Polyphagia- _____

   10. Polyuria- _____

   11. Prostaglandin- _____

   12. Puberty- _____

Just the Facts

   1. The primary function of the endocrine system is to produce ⃝ _ _ _ _ _ _ _ that
      monitor and coordinate _ _ ⃝ _ _ _ _ _ ⃝ _ _ _ _ _ _ _.

   2. Hormones are _ _ _ _ ⃝ _ _ _ _ _ _ _ _ _ _ _ _ _ _ ⃝ _ secreted
      by the endocrine glands.

   3. Three categories of hormones include _ _ _ _ _ _ hormones, _ _ _ hormones,
      and _ _ _ _ _ _ _ _ hormones.

   4. Hormones direct body processes including _ _ _ _ _ ⃝ ,
      ⃝ _ _ _ _ _ _ _ _ _ _, and _ _ _ ⃝ _ _ _ _ _ _ _ _ _
      functions.

   5. The _ ⃝ _ _ _ _ _ _ _ _ _ _ _ is a structure located above the pituitary
      gland that translates nervous system impulses into endocrine system messages.

   6. The _ _ _ _ _ ⃝ _ _ _ gland is sometimes called the "master" gland because the
      hormones that it produces regulate the secretion of other glands.

   7. The _ _ _ _ ⃝ _ _ produces hormones that regulate body metabolism.

   8. The ⃝ _ _ _ _ _ _ _ produces the hormones that regulate transportation of sugar,
      fatty acids, and amino acids into the cells

   9. Insulin dependent diabetes occurs when the pancreas secretes too little insulin resulting in
      _ ⃝ _ ⃝ _ _ _ _ _ _ _ _ _ _.

   10. Two disorders of the endocrine system that lead to an abnormal body size are
       _ _ _ _ _ _ _ _ and _ _ _ _ _ _ ⃝ _.

Use the circled letters to form the answer to this jumble. Clue: What is the disorder of the endocrine system that may lead to exophthalmos?

— — — — — — — — — — — — — — — — — — —

Concept Applications

Identifying Structures and Functions of the Endocrine System

Use Figure 17-1 in the textbook to label the diagram of the endocrine system in Figure 17-1. In the spaces provided in Table 17-1, describe the function of each part.

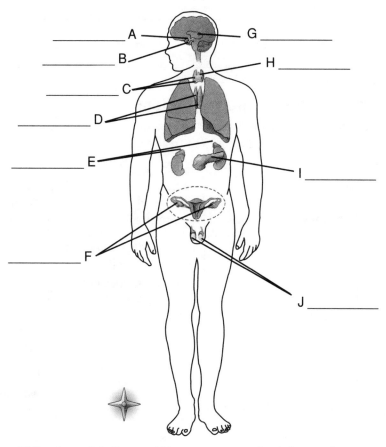

Figure 17-1 (From Thibodeau GA, Patton KT: *Anatomy & Physiology*, ed 5, St. Louis, 2003, Mosby)

TABLE 17-1

Gland	Main Function
1. Pituitary	_____
2. Pineal body	_____
3. Thyroid	_____
4. Parathyroid	_____
5. Pancreas	_____
6. Adrenal	_____
7. Ovary	_____
8. Testes	_____
9. Thymus	_____
10. Hypothalomus	_____

Identifying Disorders of the Endocrine System

Use the textbook to complete the missing information about endocrine disorders in Table 17-2. Note the etiology (causing factor), signs and symptoms, and treatment and method of prevention (if any).

TABLE 17-2

Disorder	Etiology	Signs and Symptoms	Treatment and Prevention
		Normal trunk and head with shortened extremities, does not affect intelligence	
			Removal of part or all of the thyroid
			Low-carbohydrate diet with high protein
		Women may develop male sexual characteristics	
		Polydipsia, polyuria, polyphagia	
			Administration of cortisone, decrease in sodium intake, monitoring of blood level of potassium
	Autoimmune disorder of iodine deficiency		

Applying Your Knowledge

1. Two hereditary conditions that are caused by different hormone imbalances and lead to abnormal growth and appearance are _____ and _____.

2. Two conditions that result in hyposecretion and the adrenal glands are _____ and _____.

3. A person who exhibits symptoms of frequent thirst, hunger, weight loss, and increased urine output might be tested for _____ _____.

4. Iodized salt is one method by which the hormone _____ is ensured an adequate supply of this mineral.

5. The test that determines the amount of energy needed by the body for functions of the resting body is called _____ _____ _____. A lower value in this area might indicate a problem with the _____.

Investigations

Testing Urine for Sugar and Ketone

Diabetes mellitus is a disorder of the pancreas characterized by inadequate secretion of the hormone insulin. Insulin regulates the transportation of fatty acids, sugar, and amino acids into the cells. Without insulin, sugar (glucose) cannot be used as a source of energy and fat is used instead. When fat is broken down to be used for energy, a molecule called a *ketone* is left over. Ketone is the same structure as the chemical called *acetone*. When diabetes is not controlled, the ketone and sugar molecules are carried through the blood until they are removed by the kidneys. The accuracy of the Clinitest and Acetest is very important. Medication and food needs of the diabetic client are based on the results of this simple test.

Read all of the directions before beginning this activity. Disposable gloves are worn when handling body secretions such as urine. Laboratory activities are performed only under the supervision of a qualified professional.

Urine is 95% water.

Equipment and Supplies

chemical reagent strips or pills with indicator chart
disposable gloves
test tube
urine specimen

Directions

1. Collect a fresh routine specimen of urine.

2. If pills are used to test for sugar and ketone in the urine, follow the manufacturer's instructions. The reaction of the urine and the chemical reagent in the tablet produces heat. Care must be taken to prevent burns from the test tube.

3. Strips treated with a special chemical reagent often are used to test for sugar and ketone in the urine. The reagent strip changes color when sugar or ketone is present in the urine. The degree of color change indicates the percentage of sugar or ketone in the specimen. Follow the manufacturer's instructions about the length of time to wait before comparing the reagent strip with the color chart on the bottle. Do not touch the bottle with the urine-soaked strip.

4. Dispose of the specimen, gloves, and other supplies as instructed. Make sure the laboratory area and your hands are washed thoroughly.

5. Record the results of the Clinitest for the percentage of sugar in the specimen:

   _____

6. Record the results of the Acetest for the percentage of ketones in the specimen:

   _____

Drawing Conclusions

1. Why is it important to time the exposure of the pills or strips precisely as indicated in the instructions when checking the quantity of sugar or ketone present?

   _____

   _____

   _____

2. Why is it important to avoid touching the bottle with the urine-soaked strip?

   _____

   _____

   _____

3. What household item is generally made primarily of ketone? Why do you think it might be harmful to the body for this molecule to be present in the blood?

   _____

   _____

   _____

4. If the Clinitest and Acetest indicate the presence of sugar but not fat in the urine, what do these results mean?

   _____

   _____

   _____

5. Blood also may be used to test for sugar levels. A small prick is made in the finger, and a drop of blood is placed on a testing strip made for this purpose. Which method would provide the most accurate reading on which to base the amount of insulin needed? Why is this true?

   _____

   _____

   _____

6. Compare the benefits and drawbacks of using urine or blood samples for testing sugar content of the blood.

   _____

   _____

   _____

Critical Thinking

Hormones and Adolescence

Many problems experienced by adolescents are related to hormone changes and imbalances. For example, the age of reaching puberty varies greatly among individuals. Development of secondary sexual characteristics at an early or late age may greatly influence the development of a positive self-concept. Diabetes mellitus is often discovered for the first time during adolescent years. Anorexia nervosa and steroid abuse cause changes in the function of many organs, including those of the endocrine system.

Examining the Evidence

1. What do you think would be the feelings of a boy who develops secondary sexual characteristics several years later than his peers?

   _____

   _____

   _____

2. What kind of behavior might result from this boy's feelings?

   _____

   _____

   _____

3. What do you think would be the feelings of a girl who develops secondary sexual characteristics several years earlier than her peers?

   _____

   _____

   _____

4. What kind of behavior might result from this girl's feelings?

   _____

   _____

   _____

5. Why do you think that people continue behaviors, such as abuse of steroids and eating disorders, that have been demonstrated to harm them?

   _____

   _____

   _____

6. When diabetes is discovered in an adolescent it is often difficult for the person to adjust to having the condition. Why do you think that this might be true?

   _____

   _____

   _____

Hormone Function

Hormones may be categorized according to the type of function they have in the body. These functions may stimulate other endocrine glands (tropic), reproduction (sex), or building of tissues (androgenic). Place the hormones in the chart according to their function as described in Chapter 17 of the textbook.

Thyroid-stimulating hormone	Calcitonin
Adrenocorticotropic hormone	Insulin
Follice-stimulating hormone	Thyroxine
Estrogen	Triiodothyronine
Luteinizing hormone	Prostaglandin
Interstitial cell-stimulating hormone	Progesterone
Prolactin	Androgen
Somatotropic hormone	Cortisol
Antidiuretic hormone	Aldosterone
Oxytocin	Epinephrine
Melatonin	Glucagon
Parathyroid hormone	Testosterone
Thymosin	Norepinephrine

Tropic Hormone	Sex Hormone	Anabolic Hormone
_____	_____	_____
_____	_____	_____
_____	_____	_____
_____	_____	_____
_____	_____	_____
_____	_____	_____
_____	_____	_____
_____	_____	_____
_____	_____	_____
_____	_____	_____
_____	_____	_____
_____	_____	_____

18 Nervous System

Vapid Vocabulary

Before reading the chapter, challenge your knowledge of words used in the chapter by completing the crossword puzzle of glossary terms.

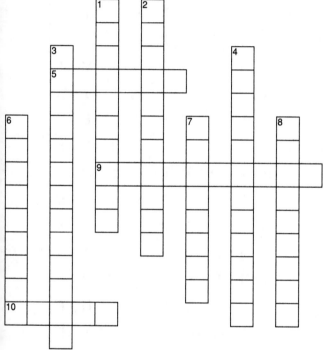

ACROSS

5 Pertaining to alternate muscular contraction and relaxation in rapid succession
9 Pertaining to the extremities or edges; away from the center
10 Having muscle tone

DOWN

1 Specialized use of radiographs to show structures in one plane of the body by blurring the image of other planes
2 State of balance
3 Neurotransmitter between muscles and nerves
4 Deterioration, change from higher to lower (less functional) form
6 A microorganism that is found temporarily
7 Neurotransmitter in central nervous system
8 Pain-reliever

Key Search

Find the Key Terms from the chapter in the word search puzzle below. Define each of the terms in the space provided.

```
D  A  I  T  M  E  M  E  D  E  P  I  L  E  P  S  Y  N  N  P
E  I  S  E  G  N  I  N  E  M  O  I  N  N  E  U  E  M  N  F
R  L  U  O  H  R  N  E  L  L  D  D  P  I  S  U  H  E  S  E
X  R  I  L  M  D  N  R  E  M  E  I  O  D  R  O  E  N  A  G
I  I  A  R  F  E  L  L  R  T  H  I  A  O  E  N  E  S  I  O
A  A  Y  O  R  L  M  I  A  T  M  N  T  P  R  F  M  E  A  I
L  H  I  T  E  I  A  R  I  N  D  R  M  O  E  R  S  L  T  E
N  T  R  M  L  E  E  N  F  N  A  I  I  O  T  P  Y  I  H  S
N  R  Y  N  E  N  I  N  I  N  H  M  Y  F  C  O  M  N  M  I
R  M  I  C  E  H  E  E  S  P  P  A  Y  E  A  O  E  E  Y  N
E  R  R  G  E  Y  C  M  Y  U  S  X  E  L  F  E  R  S  E  G
E  P  E  I  N  O  I  S  L  E  G  O  A  I  I  E  E  I  L  E
I  R  A  E  E  T  Y  S  I  I  I  E  R  O  R  R  P  E  O  M
O  E  A  P  T  A  E  L  I  E  S  M  Y  B  O  E  Y  I  G  E
R  A  A  E  O  R  E  I  I  N  R  M  E  I  E  R  E  F  R  X
A  E  R  L  A  I  N  A  R  C  A  R  T  N  I  R  O  A  A  N
P  O  L  Y  N  E  U  R  I  T  I  S  I  D  E  Y  E  N  P  E
I  T  U  L  O  A  F  N  I  A  E  R  A  Y  E  E  S  C  H  E
G  N  I  N  N  L  N  H  H  E  E  E  X  I  A  E  M  E  Y  E
A  A  R  T  E  E  E  O  U  R  E  T  D  E  E  A  T  E  E  E
```

1. Cerebrospinal fluid-_____
2. Dementia- _____
3. Epilepsy- _____
4. Impulse- _____
5. Intracranial-_____
6. Ischemia-_____
7. Meninges- _____
8. Myelography- _____
9. Neurotransmitter- _____
10. Polyneuritis- _____

11. Reflex- _____

12. Regenerate- _____

13. Senile- _____

Just the Facts

1. The function of the nervous system is to _ _ _ _ _ _,
   _ _ _ _ _ ◯ _ _ _ _, and _ _ _ _ _ _ _ _ to internal and external
   environmental changes to maintain a steady state in the body.

2. The central nervous system is made up of the _ _ ◯ _ _ and _ _ _ _ _ _ _
   _ _ _ _.

3. The peripheral nervous system consists of 12 pairs of _ _ _ _ _ _ _ nerves and 31
   pairs of _ _ _ _ _ _ nerves.

4. The _ _ _ _ _ _ _ _ ◯ _ nervous system has two parts called the sympathetic system and the parasympathetic system.

5. The basic structural unit of the nervous system is the _ _ _ _ _ that consists of
   ◯ _ _ _ _ _ cells.

6. The neuron has three main parts called the _ _ _ _ _ _ _ _ _ _, _ _ _ _,
   and _ _ _ _.

7. A ◯ _ _ _ _ _ _ is the space between two neurons.

8. The four major areas of the brain are the _ _ _ _ _ _ ◯ _ _, the diencephalon, the
   _ _ _ _ _ _ _ _ _ _, and the brain stem.

9. Two nervous system disorders that result from genetic causes are _ ◯ _ _
   _ _ _ _ _ _ _ _ and _ _ ◯ _ _ _ _ _ _ _'_ chorea.

10. The disorder of the nervous system called a transient ischemic _ _ _ _ _ ◯ may be an
    indicator for a more severe condition called a
    _ _ _ _ _ _ _ _ _ ◯ _ _ _ _ _ _ _ _ _ _ _ _ _.

Use the circled letters to form the answer to this jumble. Clue: What nervous system disorder has been treated with some success by implanting cells in the brain?

_ _ _ _ _ _ _ _ _'_

Concept Applications

Identifying Structures and Functions of the Neuron

Use Figure 18-4 in the textbook to label the diagram of the neuron in Figure 18-1. In Table 18-1, describe the function of each part.

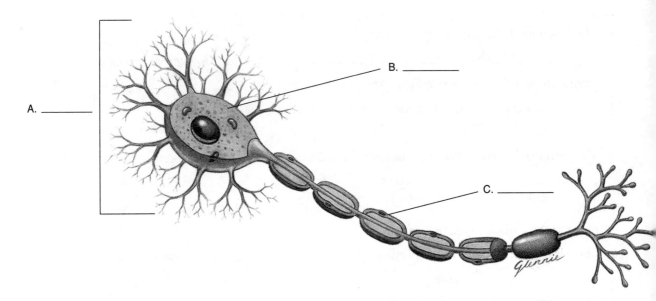

A. _____

B. _____

C. _____

Figure 18-1

TABLE 18-1

Neuron Part	Main Function
1. Axon	_____
2. Dendrite	_____
3. Cell body	_____
4. Schwann cell	_____
5. Node of Ranvier	_____

Identifying Structures and Functions of the Brain

Use Figure 18-6 in the textbook to label the diagram of the brain in Figure 18-2. In Table 18-2, describe the function of each part.

The human brain weighs 2 to 3 pounds.

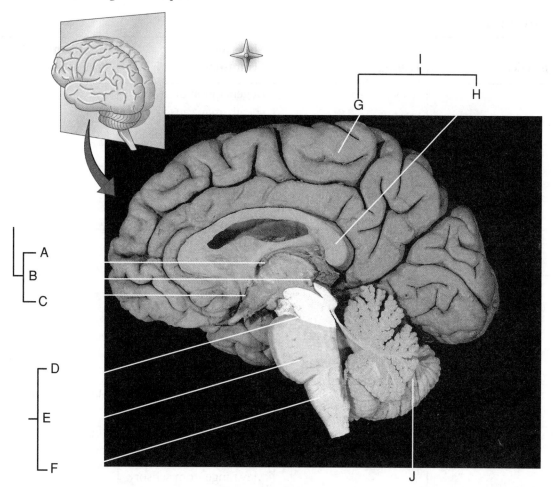

Figure 18–2 Courtesy of Thibodeau GA, Patton KT: *Anatomy and Physiology,* ed 4, St. Louis, 1999, Mosby.

TABLE 18–2

Brain Part	Main Function
1. Cerebrum	
2. Cerebellum	
3. Medulla	
4. Midbrain	
5. Temporal lobe	
6. Occipital lobe	
7. Parietal lobe	
8. Pons	
9. Frontal lobe	
10. Spinal cord	

Identifying Disorders of the Nervous System

Use the textbook to complete the missing information about nervous system disorders in Table 18-3. Note the etiology (causing factor), signs and symptoms, and treatment and method of prevention (if any).

TABLE 18-3

Disorder	Etiology	Signs and Symptoms	Treatment and Prevention
		Degeneration of myelin sheath, may cause double vision or loss of muscle control	
	Blood clot or vessel break causes ischemia in brain		
		Paralysis below the area of injury	
		Loss of memory and progressive impaired function	
	Bacteria, virus, or fungus		
			May require prescription medicine, may be triggered by certain foods
		May range from sensory change to loss of responsiveness with tonic/clonic movement	

Applying Your Knowledge

1. One of the most common forms of mental retardation results from a genetic disorder that is caused by the presence of an extra chromosome. This condition is called _____

   _____.

2. When the brain is damaged by lack of oxygen in one area, the condition may commonly be called a _____.

3. Head pains due to stress are called _____ headaches, whereas those that result from vascular problems of unknown cause are called _____. Swelling of membranes in the skull's cavities may lead to a third kind called _____ headaches.

4. Prenatal testing during the 14th to 16th week of pregnancy may be used to determine whether a defect in spinal development of the embryo is present. This condition may be called a

_____   _____   _____.

5. One neurological disorder that may be prevented by vaccination is _____.

Investigations

Assessing Neurologic Signs

One method used to quickly determine the level of function of the neurologic system is to assess the neurologic vital signs or "neuro" signs. The following is the procedure for a short assessment of these functions. Read all of the directions before beginning this activity. Laboratory activities should be completed only under the supervision of a qualified professional.

Equipment and Supplies

penlight

Directions

1. Work in pairs for this activity. One person acts as subject and the other as examiner throughout the activity. The roles may then be reversed.

2. Construct a chart to record the information needed to document the results of this activity. Place each type of assessment in the vertical column and "Right," "Left," and "Comments" as the horizontal column titles.

3. Observe the subject to determine the level of responsiveness. Level of responsiveness may be described in one of the following terms:
   - alert: aware of surroundings and environmental stimuli; responds to verbal stimulus such as talking
   - lethargic: may be made aware of environmental stimuli with assistance; responds to loud verbal stimuli or touch.
   - stuporous: does not respond to environmental stimuli; may be roused with return to sleepwalk state quickly; responds to touch and pain stimuli
   - comatose: does not respond to any stimuli
   Record the level of responsiveness of the subject being examined:

   _____

4. Determine the orientation of the subject by asking questions that assess awareness of person, place, and time. Questions should require more than a yes or no answer to determine if the answer is appropriate. For example:
   "Tell me your name please" asks for orientation of person. It would be acceptable for the person to name a relative if asked for that information.
   "What day of the week is it?" asks for orientation to time. This question may be difficult for someone who has been hospitalized for a while. Knowing the year or the name of the current president would be acceptable in this and some other circumstances.
   "Tell me the name of this facility" asks for orientation to place. Knowing the city or similar information would be acceptable in these and some other situations.

Normal orientation is "oriented × 3" or to all three areas of inquiry. If the person being examined is not oriented in one or more of the areas, an example of the incorrect response should be recorded. If the subject cannot answer or gives incorrect responses, the correct information should be given to the subject to prevent anxiety.
Record the orientation of the subject:

5. Assess the response of the pupils to light. Observe the pupils of both eyes. They should be equal in size. Turn on a small flashlight or penlight. Bring the light from the side of the face to shine into the center of the subject's right eye, keeping the flashlight about 6 inches away from the face. Observe the pupils of both eyes as the light nears the right eye. The pupils of both eyes should contract quickly and equally. Remove the light. The pupils should return to their original size quickly and equally. Repeat the exercise by shining the light in the left eye. This result is recorded as PEERL or PERRLA (pupils equal in size and equally reactive to light).
Record the results of the pupil responses:

_____

6. Assess the function of facial nerves and muscles. Instruct the subject to stick out the tongue as far as possible. The tongue should extend in a symmetrical manner on both sides.
Record the results of the facial muscle response:

_____

7. Assess the strength and equality of nerve and muscle response of the hands. Instruct the subject to grip and squeeze the index and middle finger of both of the examiner's hands as hard as possible until asked to stop. The grips of the subject should be equal and strong.
Record the results of the grip responses:

_____

8. Assess the strength and equality of the nerve and muscle response of the feet. For this assessment, the subject should be lying down or sitting with the legs extended. The examiner places one arm across the soles of the subject's feet and instructs the subject to push as hard as possible with both feet. The push response of the subject's feet should be equal and strong.
Record the results of the push responses:

_____

Drawing Conclusions

1. When neurologic vital signs are taken every 15 minutes, it is necessary to vary the questions slightly. It is also important to explain to the client that the procedure will be repeated. What might the client think if the procedure were repeated several times without explanation?

_____

_____

_____

2. Clients are given more than one chance to answer questions of orientation correctly. This is especially important if the client is awakened for the assessment. Why would this be important?

_____

_____

_____

3. A person may have a level of responsiveness of being alert and an orientation of being confused. How would this appear in the neurologic assessment?

_____

_____

_____

4. Which cranial nerve is being assessed when the pupil resonse is tested?

_____

_____

_____

5. Why is it necessary to test the pupil response by shining the light into each eye separately?

_____

_____

_____

6. List three factors that might influence the results of this assessment.

_____

_____

_____

Assessing Cranial Nerve Functions

One of the methods used to assess neurologic function tests the function of the cranial nerves. Use the textbook to list each of the 12 cranial nerves and their functions in Table 18-4. Then complete the laboratory activity. Read all of the directions before begining this activity. Laboratory activities should be completed only under the supervision of a qualified professional.

TABLE 18-4

Cranial Nerve	Main Function
I. _____	_____
II. _____	_____
III. _____	_____
IV. _____	_____
V. _____	_____
VI. _____	_____
VII. _____	_____
VIII. _____	_____
IX. _____	_____
X. _____	_____
XI. _____	_____
XII. _____	_____

Equipment and Supplies

alarm clock
audiogram (optional)
containers of items for identification of odor
cotton swabs
items for assessment of taste
penlight
Snellen chart
tongue depressor

Directions

1. Work in pairs for this activity. One person acts as subject and the other as examiner throughout the activity. The roles may then be reversed.

2. Construct a chart on which to record the results of this activity.

3. To assess the function of the first cranial nerve, the subject to be examined closes both eyes and blocks one nostril. The examiner presents items for identification that have a familiar odor. Items to be smelled should be kept in sealed containers before and after use. Some examples of items for identification include coffee, soap, peanut butter, and vanilla. Repeat the process for the other nostril.
   Record the results of the assessment:

   _____

4. The second cranial nerve can be tested using an eye chart to determine visual acuity. The procedure for determining visual acuity is presented in Chapter 24 of the textbook.
   Record the visual acuity of each eye separately and both eyes together:

   _____

5. The third, fourth, and sixth cranial nerves can be tested at the same time because they all regulate eye movement. The subject may demonstrate this function by following the movement of the examiner's finger in lateral and vertical directions. Eye movement should be the same with both eyes.
   Record the results of the assessment:

   _____

6. The motor function of the fifth cranial nerve can be assessed with the subject biting down on the teeth as hard as possible. The muscles of the jaw should be observed to be tight and equal in size. The sensory function of this nerve can be assessed for the equal sensation of temperature and touch on both sides of the face.
   Record the results of the assessment:

   _____

7. The seventh cranial nerve has both sensory and motor function. The motor function controls facial expression. To assess this nerve, the subject frowns, smiles widely, and puffs out the cheeks. The muscle movements should appear equal in strength and symmetry. The procedure for assessing the sensory or taste function of this nerve is presented in Chapter 19 of the workbook.
   Record the results of the assessment:

   _____

8. The eighth cranial nerve can be assessed using the audiogram to perform a hearing test. The function may also be assessed in a rough manner by using a small winding alarm clock. The ticking noise of the clock should be heard by the subject when 20 feet from it. Test each ear separately by blocking one at a time and then both together for the assessment.
Record the results of the assessment:

_____

9. The ninth and tenth cranial nerves may be assessed at the same time. Part of the function of the ninth cranial nerve is taste on the posterior tongue. It may be tested in the manner described in Chapter 19 of the workbook. However, swallowing and the gag reflex demonstrate the motor functionof these nerves. When an object touches the posterior pharynx, the palate should elevate and retract upward. A clean tongue depressor may be used with care to prevent injury to the soft tissues of the mouth for this assessment.
Record the results of the assessment:

_____

10. The eleventh cranial nerve activates the movement of the trapezius and sternocleidomastoid muscles. This function is assessed by having the subject turn the head to one side and push the chin in the same direction against the resistance of the examiner's hand. The sternocleidomastoid muscle in the neck should stand out visibly with this effort. The trapezius muscle can be assessed in the same manner by shrugging or lifting the shoulders against the examiner's hands on the shoulders. The force of the resistance against the examiner's hands should be strong.
Record the results of the assessment:

_____

11. The twelfth cranial nerve may be assessed by observing the movement of the tongue. The subject sticks the tongue out. The tongue should extend in a symmetrical manner.
Record the results of the assessment:

_____

Drawing Conclusions

1. Why must the assessments be performed separately for both sides of the body?

_____

_____

_____

2. In the assessment of the olfactory nerve, why is it important to keep the containers sealed tightly before and after being used for assessment?

_____

_____

_____

3. Why is it necessary to test both the motor and sensory function of the trigeminal, facial, glossopharyngeal, and vagus cranial nerves?

_____

_____

_____

4. Are the results of the assessment within the normal range?

_____

_____

_____

5. List three factors that might influence the results of this activity.

_____

_____

_____

Critical Thinking

Coma Therapy

Sensory stimulation is used with great success to treat people in comas. Some examples of stimulation include the use of loud music and application of hot peppers and vinegar on the tongue. Ammonia is used to activate the sense of smell. Conversation is held in the room and directed to the comatose individual to stimulate the brain's responses. This type of aggressive coma therapy is based on the theory that continual stimulation of the senses helps the brain remember these stimulants and how to respond to them. With aggressive therapy, coma clients receive 8 hours of intensive activity each day, including physical, occupational, and speech therapy.

Examining the Evidence

1. The cost of intensive coma therapy is high. How do you think this cost might compare with the cost of maintaining someone in a coma for a long period of time?

_____

_____

_____

2. The theory behind aggressive stimulation of the senses for a comatose client assumes that the brain is able to assess and respond to stimuli even if no reaction is seen. Describe at least one other situation or state in which a person is normally unresponsive to stimuli.

_____

_____

_____

3. If the theory about the brain's responses is proven to be true, how might that alter the care of the client in the state you described in question two?

_____

_____

_____

Recognizing Reflexes

Fill in Table 18-5 by indicating the reflex that occurs as a result of the indicated stimulus.

TABLE 18-5

Stimulus	Reflex Action that Results
1. Feeling cold and wet	
2. Feeling hot	
3. Coming up after swimming underwater	
4. Swallowing into the trachea	
5. Loud, unexpected noise	
6. Getting a foreign particle in the eye	
7. Inhaling pepper	
8. Bright light	
9. Being tickled	
10. Stepping on a tack	

19 Sensory System

Vapid Vocabulary

Before reading the chapter, challenge your knowledge of words used in the chapter by completing the crossword puzzle of glossary terms.

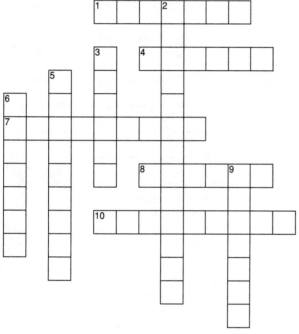

ACROSS

1 Of a fatty nature, fat
4 Evenly curved, resembling part of a sphere
7 Situated entirely within or pertaining exclusively to a part
8 Sharpness or clearness
10 Any small mass or body

DOWN

2 Receptor that responds to stimulus originating in the body itself, especially to pressure, position, and stretching
3 Substance that transmits impulses or that serves as growth location for microorganisms
5 Coming from or originating outside
6 Organic material that gives color in the body
9 Pertaining to the touch

Key Search

Find the Key Terms from the chapter in the word search puzzle below. Define each of the terms in the space provided.

```
O  N  O  S  S  E  E  C  O  S  D  M  A  E  I  I  I  E  A  E
T  T  A  U  U  E  O  E  T  E  R  O  G  Q  O  E  S  C  D  E
R  S  S  C  L  U  T  N  E  E  T  L  R  U  C  T  U  T  S  U
N  N  N  R  U  C  R  S  U  S  A  S  O  I  I  S  E  U  O  T
A  C  C  O  M  M  O  D  A  T  I  O  N  L  V  C  R  S  N  A
S  U  A  C  I  S  A  Y  S  S  R  G  R  I  I  I  Y  A  M  L
A  T  Y  D  T  T  O  R  U  O  U  A  O  B  S  R  R  S  Y  T
I  I  R  R  S  T  C  O  M  S  A  T  O  R  I  O  O  R  R  R
I  T  A  O  Y  E  E  A  T  I  E  N  E  I  O  E  O  O  Y  G
E  M  G  T  S  N  G  A  R  T  E  I  C  U  N  T  R  N  R  O
E  U  O  I  A  A  T  R  G  F  U  E  L  M  C  T  N  S  O  G
U  M  G  T  S  O  T  S  E  S  E  O  M  A  O  U  Y  O  T  T
C  R  U  E  R  U  T  E  S  V  U  R  F  O  I  O  D  A  I  U
S  C  R  Y  O  L  O  T  M  T  N  L  L  O  S  U  C  Y  D  C
G  M  G  Y  S  T  T  L  V  A  O  O  U  R  L  O  E  R  U  R
E  O  U  R  R  T  N  T  E  C  A  U  C  S  R  U  L  F  A  E
I  N  T  R  A  O  C  U  L  A  R  O  T  S  L  Y  R  S  R  C
L  A  B  Y  R  I  N  T  H  I  U  T  I  E  I  O  L  T  H  S
N  U  T  R  G  A  I  N  I  M  T  T  A  R  O  E  C  O  I  N
R  E  C  E  P  T  O  R  I  Y  T  F  Y  R  R  I  M  R  R  T
```

1. Accommodation- _____

2. Auditory- _____

3. Converge- _____

4. Cutaneous- _____

5. Equilibrium- _____

6. Gustatory- _____

7. Intraocular- _____

8. Labyrinth- _____

9. Olfactory- _____

10. Receptor- _____

11. Refraction-_____

12. Stimulus-_____

13. Vision- _____

Just the Facts

1. The sensory system consists of receptors in specialized cells and organs that perceive changes in the _ _ _ _ _ _ _ _ _ and _ _ O_ _ _ _ _ _ environment.

2. Specialized cells called _ _ _ O_ and O_ _ _ _ _ in the retina absorb the light.

3. The _ _ _ O_ _ _ _ _ sense is the primary function of the ear, and a second function is to help maintain _ _ _ _ _ _ _ _ _ _ _ _ _.

4. Specialized cells located in _ _ _ O_ _ _ _ _ _ _ _ on the tongue or O_ _ _ _ _ _ _ _ _ _ _ _ _ _ _ _ perceive taste.

5. The olfactory sense originates in cells in the nose that immediately transmit impulses to the brain through the olfactory _ _ _ O_ _ _ _ _ _ _ _ _ O_ _ _.

6. The _ O_ _ _ _ _ _ _ _ senses of the skin perceive touch, pressure, temperature, and pain through _ O_ _ _ specialized cells located in the skin.

7. A disorder of the sensory system that is often related to diabetes mellitus is _ _ _ _ _ _ _ _ _ _ _ _ _ _ O_ _ _ _ _ _ _.

8. Two conditions of the eye that are often corrected with glasses are _ _ _ _ _ _ _ O_ _ and _ _ _ _ _ _ _.

9. A common disorder of vision that occurs with aging is _ _ _ _ _ _ _ O_ _ _ _.

10. Most people do not notice a loss in hearing until they cannot understand _ _ _ _ _ _ _ _ _ _ _ _ _ _ _ O_ _ _.

Use the circled letters to form the answer to this jumble. Clue: What is a common bacterial or viral eye infection that causes reddening of the eyelids and is extremely contagious?

_ _ _ _ _ _ _ _ _ _ _ _ _ _

Concept Applications

Identifying Structures and Functions of the Eye

Use Figure 19-1 in the textbook to label the diagram of the eye in Figure 19-1. In the spaces provided in Table 19-1, describe the function of each part.

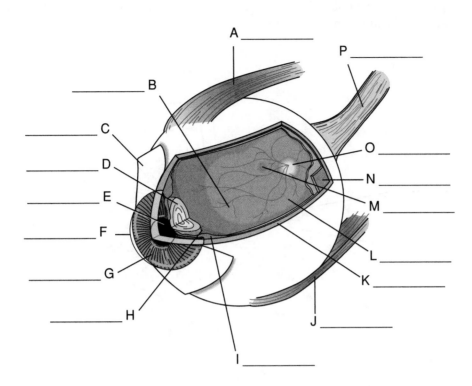

Figure 19-1 Courtesy of Sorrentino: *Mosby's Textbook for Nursing Assistants,* ed 5, Hanover, 2000, Mosby.

Only one fifth of the eye is actually exposed to the outside environment.

TABLE 19-1

Eye Part	Main Function
1. Iris	
2. Anterior cavity	
3. Pupil	
4. Cornea	
5. Lens	
6. Suspensory ligaments	
7. Sclera	
8. Choroid coat	
9. Retina	
10. Optic nerve	
11. Posterior cavity	
12. Conjuctiva	
13. Ciliary muscle	

Identifying Structures and Functions of the Ear

Use Figure 19-3 in the textbook to label the diagram of the ear in Figure 19-2. In the spaces provided in Table 19-2, describe the function of each part.

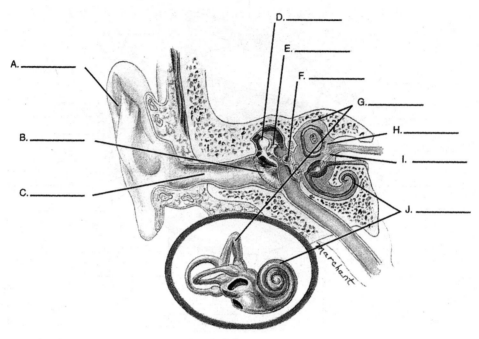

Figure 19-2 Courtesy of Sorrentino: *Mosby's Textbook for Nursing Assistants,* ed 5, Hanover, 2000, Mosby.

TABLE 19-2

Ear Part	Main Function
1. Malleus	
2. Pinna	
3. Auditory canal	
4. Tympanic membrane	
5. Oval window	
6. Stapes	
7. Cochlea	
8. Incus	
9. Semicircular canal	
10. Vestibule	

Identifying Structures and Functions of the Nose

Use Figure 19-5 in the textbook to label the diagram of the nose in Figure 19-3. In the spaces provided in Table 19-3, describe the function of each part.

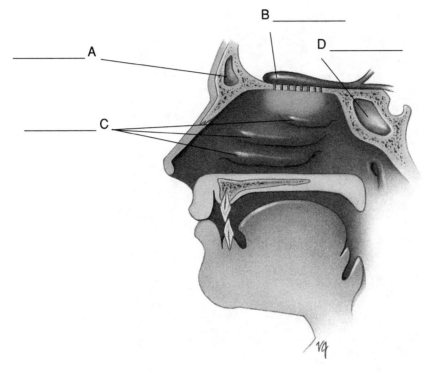

Figure 19-3

TABLE 19-3

Nose Part	Main Function
1. Frontal sinus	
2. Olfactory bulb	
3. Nasal turbinate	
4. Sphenoid sinus	

Identifying Structures and Functions of the Skin

Use Figure 19-6 in the textbook to label the diagram of the skin in Figure 19-4. In the spaces provided in Table 19-4, describe the function of each part.

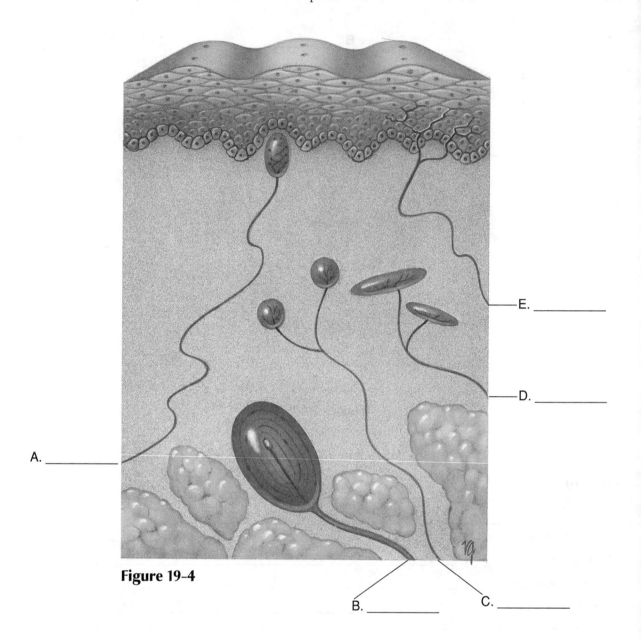

Figure 19-4

E. _____

D. _____

A. _____

B. _____

C. _____

TABLE 19-4

Skin Part	Main Function
1. Pacinian corpusles	_____
2. End–bulb of Krause	_____
3. Ruffini's corpuscles	_____
4. Pain receptor	_____
5. Meissner's corpuscles	_____

Identifying Disorders of the Sensory System

Use the textbook to complete the missing information about sensory system disorders in Table 19-5. Note the etiology (causing factor), signs and symptoms, and treatment and method of prevention (if any).

TABLE 19-5

Disorder	Etiology	Signs and Symptoms	Treatment and Prevention
			Antibiotics, may include myringotomy
	Genetic, defect on X chromosome		
		Increased intraocular pressure, may cause pain or no symptoms	
	Congenital defect of eyeball		
	Inflammation of cavity of the cranium, nasal obstruction		
		Clouding of lens of the eye leading to blurred or partial vision	
		Inflammation and reddening of eyelids and sclera with pus formation, extremely contagious	

Applying Your Knowledge

1. Hearing loss may result from a problem in _____ or _____.

2. The correct term for a nosebleed is _____. One cause may be

   _____.

3. Children with the infection called _____ _____ may be
   treated by the insertion of tubes to drain the middle ear.

4. One symptom that may be caused by sinus, chemical, viral, or allergic irritation may be

   _____.

5. A stye is caused by a bacterial infection in the _____ _____
   of the eyelid.

Investigations

Identifying Taste Receptor Locations

Read all of the directions before beginning this activity. Laboratory activities should be completed only under the supervision of a qualified professional.

Equipment and Supplies

containers of unknown liquids
disposable cotton swabs or toothpicks and cotton batting

Directions

1. Cover both tips of six toothpicks with a small wad of cotton.

2. Occlude the nose during taste testing to prevent smelling the unknown liquids.

3. Dip one end of a toothpick in the first unknown liquid and rub the swab lightly over both sides of the tongue. Record the number of the unknown liquid in the appropriate location on the diagram of the tongue in Figure 19-5 if it is tasted.

4. Dip the unused end of the same toothpick in the first unknown liquid and rub the swab lightly over the tip and back of the tongue. Record the number of the unknown liquid in the appropriate location on the diagram of the tongue if tasted.

5. Discard the toothpick in the proper location. Using a new toothpick for each unknown liquid, repeat the procedure for each of the other liquids.

Drawing Conclusions

1. In this activity, care is taken to prevent dipping the part of the toothpick that has been placed in the subject's mouth back into the unknown liquids. Why would this be important?

   _____

   _____

   _____

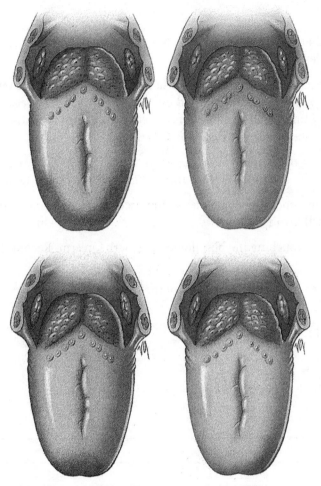

Figure 19-5

2. Obtain a list of the contents of the unknown liquids. Label your diagram with the types of liquids next to the location where they were tasted. Note if the locations are consistent with the locations for taste identified in the textbook. Why might these results be different?

   _____

   _____

   _____

3. Why are the nostrils occluded throughout this activity?

   _____

   _____

   _____

Demonstrating Skin Sensitivity

Although receptors for touch are located on all surfaces of the body, the type and frequency of these receptors vary. Read all of the directions before beginning this activity. Laboratory activities should be completed only under the supervision of a qualified professional.

Equipment and Supplies

blindfold
bristles of varied size

Directions

1. Work in pairs for this activity. One person acts as subject and the other as examiner throughout the activity. The roles may then be reversed.

2. The smallest stimulus that produces a response of a neuron is called the *threshold stimulus*. To determine the threshold stimulus, blindfold one of the partners. The second person gently touches the fingertip of the blindfolded partner with a small bristle until it bends. The blindfolded partner tells the examiner if the bristle can be felt.

3. Repeat step one using three different bristles of varied thicknesses. Try each bristle randomly, using each type at least five times. Record the rsults of the activity in Table 19-6.

4. Repeat the procedure touching the bristles to the back of the blindfolded partner's hand. Record the results of this activity in Table 19-7.

5. Repeat the procedure touching the blindfolded partner's forearm. Record the results of this activity in Table 19-8.

6. Repeat the procedure by touching the back of the blindfolded partner's neck with the bristles. Record the results of this activity in Table 19-9.

7. Exchange roles and repeat the activity.

Drawing Conclusions

1. Which part of the body tested has the lowest threshold of sensitivity (which felt the thinnest bristle most frequently)?

   _____

   _____

   _____

2. Which part of the body tested has the highest threshold of sensitivity (which felt the thinnest bristles least frequently?

   _____

   _____

   _____

3. Based on your observations, hypothesize why some areas of the skin are more sensitive than others.

   _____

   _____

   _____

TABLE 19-6 Fingertip

Bristle	SM	MED	LG
Trial 1			
Trial 2			
Trial 3			
Trial 4			
Trial 5			

TABLE 19-7 Back of Hand

Bristle	SM	MED	LG
Trial 1			
Trial 2			
Trial 3			
Trial 4			
Trial 5			

TABLE 19-8 Forearm

Bristle	SM	MED	LG
Trial 1			
Trial 2			
Trial 3			
Trial 4			
Trial 5			

TABLE 19-9 Back of Neck

Bristle	SM	MED	LG
Trial 1			
Trial 2			
Trial 3			
Trial 4			
Trial 5			

Critical Thinking

Patterns of Sleep

About one third of a human life is spent sleeping. Sleeping is defined as the recurrent, normal condition of unresponsiveness with limited movement. Scientists do not agree on the reason that sleep occurs, but all agree that is is necessary for a healthy life. The theories that have been suggested to explain the need for sleep include:

- to remove buildup of metabolic waste from the brain
- to allow rest of the nerve tissues
- to remove excess hormones from the body

Research into sleep patterns and disorders is a relatively new field. The time spent sleeping has been divided into five stages based on the brain's wave patterns. Drawsiness or relaxed wakefulness precedes but is not considered part of sleep. During this time the brain produces alpha waves, and images may occur in the brain. These images are not considered dreams. The stages of sleep are found in Table 19-10.

TABLE 19-10

Stage	Description	Brain Wave Pattern	Length	% of Sleep
Stage 1	Lightest sleep	Reduced alpha	1–2 min	
Stage 2	Light sleep	Frequent, regular waves	5–10 min	50%
Stage 3		Transition to delta waves	10 min	
Stage 4	Deep sleep	Delta brain waves	5–15 min	
Stage 5	REM or dream sleep		45 min	20%–25%

Normally, a person passes through the stages of sleep several times during a sleep cycle. At the end of each cycle, the brain wave activity resembles light sleep and rapid eye movement (REM) can be observed. This part of sleep is called *dream sleep*. The first period of REM sleep is the shortest with each period becoming longer. The REM stage may be as long as 45 minutes in length before waking occurs. Whether the dreams are remembered or not, every person has three to five REM periods each night.

The amount of sleep necessary varies between individuals. Generally newborns and infants need 14 to 20 hours of sleep. Young children need 12 to 14 hours of sleep. Adults usually need 7 to 9 hours in each 24-hour period. Sleep deprivation leads to a decrease in performance, irritability, agitation, tremors, lack of attention, and lethargy. Over a long period, lack of sleep can lead to brain damage and death. Sleep disorders are called *parasomnias*. The following is a description of several types of sleep patterns.

Insomnia is the inability to sleep. It is usually a symptom of another disorder. Insomniacs fall into three categories: some people have difficulty falling asleep, others have trouble staying asleep, and other insomniacs wake early. Generally, insomnia is caused by overstimulation due to anxiety, stress, or stimulants.

Hypersomnia is the condition in which a person sleeps 16 to 18 hours a day. This condition may be acute or chronic in nature. It often occurs with uremia, increased intracranial pressure, diabetic acidosis, or hypothyroidism. It may also occur as a reaction to stress.

Sleep apnea is a disorder that most often occurs in middle-aged men who are overweight and have high blood pressure. The person experiencing sleep apnea generally snores and then stops breathing for 30 to 40 seconds. It is believed that the epiglottis falls back into the throat closing the airway. The condition can be life threatening.

Enuresis, or bed wetting, has no clear-cut cause. Restricting fluid intake several hours before sleeping helps control the condition.

Somnambulism is commonly called *sleep walking*. It is seen most often in children, who eventually outgrow it. People who are sleep walking are easily awakened and are not dreaming during this stage of sleep.

Almost everyone talks while asleep at some time.

Bruxism is teeth grinding that occurs during sleep. This condition may cause discomfort and damage to teeth. Appliances or mouth guards may be worn to protect the teeth.

Night terrors and nightmares may become a serious sleep disorder. The autonomic nervous system actually produces stress responses in the body during night terrors.

Narcolepsy is a form of epilepsy in which sleep occurs regardless of position or activity. It is commonly called a *sleep attack*. Narcolepsy may often be controlled with medication.

Sleep may be induced with drugs that include sedatives. Sedatives, alcohol, tranquilizers, hypnotics, and amphetamines are drugs that alter the sleep pattern. When one of these drugs has been taken on a regular basis, rebound nightmares will occur when the drug is stopped. It takes 3 to 5 weeks for the sleep cycle to return to normal once it has been altered.

Examining the Evidence

1. How much sleep is needed by a person in adolescence?

   _____

   _____

   _____

2. List five signs and symptoms that may indicate an inadequate amount of sleep.

   _____

   _____

   _____

3. Why is sleep apnea life threatening?

   _____

   _____

   _____

Issues of Hearing Loss

Normally, the human ear can distinguish or separate more than 350,000 different sounds. It is the most complex and efficient sensory organ. In the United States, hearing loss is the fourth most prevalent chronic physical disability. About one in eight Americans will suffer some hearing loss during a lifetime.

Examining the Evidence

1. List three ways in which an adolescent's life would be altered if a serious hearing loss occurred.

   _____

   _____

   _____

2. List three methods that might be used to help someone with a serious hearing loss understand procedures during a health examination or treatment.

   _____

   _____

   _____

3. List three methods that might be used to preserve hearing later in life.

   _____

   _____

   _____

20 Reproductive System

Vapid Vocabulary

Before reading the chapter, challenge your knowledge of words used in the chapter by completing the crossword puzzle of glossary terms.

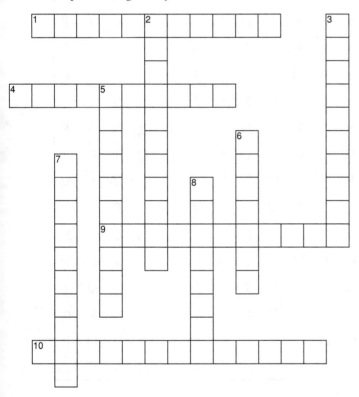

ACROSS

1 Containing blood vessels or indicative of a large blood supply
4 Agent that inhibits the growth of fungus
9 Enlargement or overgrowth of an organ or part caused by an increase in its cells
10 Agent that prevents conception or pregnancy

DOWN

2 Examination of the internal organs of the abdomen using a scope
3 Quality or condition of being able to stretch and resume original shape
5 Spiral bacteria, microorganism
6 Fill to capacity
7 Lengthening of an object
8 Plant or animal that lives on or within another living organism at the expense of the host organism

Key Search

Find the Key Terms from the chapter in the word search puzzle below. Define each of the terms in the space provided.

```
N C P C N O I T A L U V O T L E I G T N
O E I G M O Y T I L I R E T S C E V N O
I F C R E A I N R C I I C O E N R T T T
T S N T N O M T U I P S A S I I R O I C
A E F O L L I M A C L N U T M N I N C R
T S I E T C T M O T R I A C S M E L E V
C R C T I Y D E N G S L O P T Y D C T P
A U C F F C R N Y E R E C T I L E T Y C
L O A C S I L S C R M A G S F S I I M C
C C I O V O B T U F L C P C C I P S I P
L R R C A Y C R S N E U N H L L E N A R
N E C V C V I U O O O R L C Y C O T C I
Y T Y O T C C A L I S M T Y C I E Y L M
F N L C S Y O L C C D M O I T O M C Y U
Y I C C R P U C M T T O G P L P M U C N
S E S N E M L Y C V M R E N E I I I C M
T R R H R C C C N I C C I C F C T O M I
R L M N O T R L C L N R P N F P M Y R C
C I P O T C E E O O C L R C L C T L O P
U C Y A M E P C C R M C N R R O G A C L
```

1. Conception-_____

2. Ectopic- _____

3. Erectile- _____

4. Fertility-_____

5. Fibroid- _____

6. Genital- _____

7. Gestation- _____

8. Intercourse- _____

9. Lactation-_____

10. Mammography-_____

11. Menses- _____

12. Menstrual cycle- _____

13. Ovulation-_____

14. Sterility-_____

Just the Facts

1. The function of the reproductive system is to produce _ _ _ _ _ ◯ _ _ _.

2. The reproductive organs of both the male and female produce sex cells called
   _ _ ◯ _ _ _ _

3. The _ _ _ _ _ _ ◯ _ _ _ _ _ _ _ _ _ transport the mature ovum from
   the ovary to the uterus.

4. The _ _ _ _ _ _ ◯ is implanted in the uterus after conception

5. Growth of an offspring in the uterus lasts about _ _ _ _ _ _ _ ◯ (9 months), or
   through the period of pregnancy.

6. A baby born before the 37th week of pregnancy is considered to be
   ◯ _ _ _ _ _ _ _ _.

7. Many abnormalities of the breasts and testes may be discovered by
   ◯ _ _ _ - _ ◯ _ _ _ _ _ _ _ _ _ _.

8. Tests that can be used to detect abnormalities of the fetus during gestation include
   _ _ _ _ _ _ _ ◯ _ _ _ _ _ _ _, ultrasonography, and
   _ ◯ _ _ _ _ _ _ _ villus sampling.

9. Three sexually transmitted diseases that are caused by bacteria are
   _ _ ◯ _ _ _ _ ◯ _, syphilis, and _ _ _ _ _ _ _ _ _ _.

10. A common cause of _ _ _ ◯ _ _ _ _ _ _ _ is damage to the fallopian tubes
    as a result of pelvic inflammatory disease.

Use the circled letters to form the answer to this jumble. Clue: What is a common disorder of the reproductive system that results from a viral infection and has no cure?

_ _ _ _ _ _ _ _ _ _ _ _ _

Concept Applications

Identifying Structures and Functions of the Male Reproductive System

Use Figure 20-2 in the textbook to label the diagram of the male reproductive system in Figure 20-1. In the spaces provided in Table 20-1, describe the function of each part.

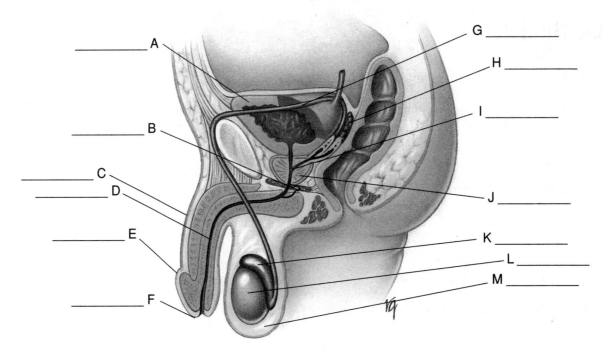

Figure 20-1

TABLE 20-1

Reproductive Part	Main Function
1. Prostate gland	
2. Urinary meatus	
3. Urinary bladder	
4. Epididymis	
5. Urethra	
6. Penis	
7. Scrotum	
8. Seminal vesicle	
9. Cowper's gland	
10. Vas deferens	
11. Testis	
12. Ejaculatory duct	
13. Glans penis	

Identifying Structures and Functions of the the Female Reproductive System

Use Figure 20-4A to B in the textbook to label the diagram of the female reproductive system in Figure 20-2A to B. In the spaces provided in Table 20-2, describe the function of each part.

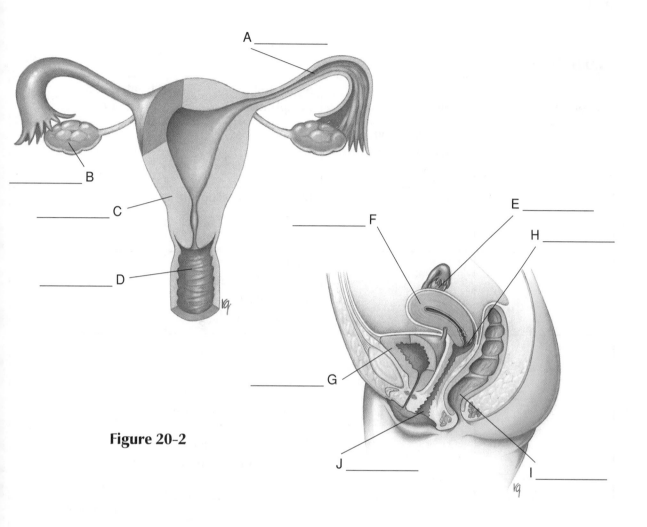

Figure 20-2

TABLE 20–2

Reproductive Part	Main Function
1. Uterus	
2. Ovary	
3. Rectum	
4. Cervix	
5. Urinary bladder	
6. Vagina	
7. Fallopian tube	

Identifying Disorders of the Reproductive System

Use the textbook to complete the missing information about reproductive system disorders in Table 20-3. Note the etiology (causing factor), signs and symptoms, and treatment and method of prevention (if any).

TABLE 20-3

Disorder	Etiology	Signs and Symptoms	Treatment and Prevention
	Chronic infection such as gonorrhea or chlamydia		
		Blisters that develop into open painful sores appearing in episodes	
		Painless sores, fever, swollen glands, rash, nervous system damage in third stage	
	Alcohol consumption by mother of unborn baby		
		Painful urination, white to yellowish green discharge from urethra, may have no symptoms in women	
			Surgical removal; freezing, chemical or electrical burning
	Hormonal or biochemical imbalance, poor nutrition		

Applying Your Knowledge

1. The most common sexually transmitted disease, called _____, is one of several that may have no symptoms in women. Another that may have no symptoms in women is called _____.

2. The child that will be affected by erythroblastosis fetalis is the _____ or later.

3. The ratio of people who develop genital warts after contact with them is _____.

4. When a mother drinks alcohol during pregnancy the effects on the fetus may be mental or physical. The condition called _____ _____

_____ can be cured by _____.

5. It is estimated that more than 100,000 women become infertile each year by the condition called

_____ _____ _____. This condition is

developed by _____ women annually.

Investigations

Demonstrating Embryo Development

Embryonic development begins after fertilization. Developmental changes in the embryo follow a set pattern to become the complex organs and tissues of the organism. Chick embryos are often used to observe embryonic development because they develop outside the mother's body. Read all of the directions before beginning this activity. Laboratory activities are completed only under the supervision of a qualified professional.

Equipment and Supplies

culture dish
dissecting scissors
eyedropper
fertilized chicken eggs
forceps
hand lens or dissecting microscope
incubator
paper towel
ruler
0.9% saline solution
unfertilized egg
vials of 70% alcohol (optional)

Directions

1. Place fertilized eggs into an incubator at 38°C for 2 days.

2. Pour a 0.9% saline solution into a culture dish until it is half full. Break an unfertilized egg open into the dish by striking the middle of the egg on the side of the dish. Observe and draw the internal organization of an unfertilized egg. Identify the albumen, yolk, and shell of the egg.

3. Gently crack open a fertilized, unincubated egg in the same manner. Observe the contents. Identify the albumen, yolk, and shell of the egg. Identify the chalaza that attaches the yolk to the center of the egg. Identify the blastoderm or small white spot on the surface of the yolk that becomes the embryo. Record the diameter of the blastoderm in millimeters: _____

4. Place a piece of crumpled paper towel in a culture dish to cushion a fertilized egg during observation. Place a mark on the top side of an egg that has been incubated for 2 days at 38°C. Move the egg from the incubator to the culture dish with the mark remaining on the top.

5. Using pointed scissors and forceps, carefully remove an oval-shaped piece of the shell from the top of the egg. If the embryo is not on the top of the yolk, gently rotate the yolk with an eyedropper until it is visible. The dropper may be used to remove the albumen for better examination of the embryo structures. Examine the embryo with a hand lens or dissecting microscope. Identify the head, brain, and blood vessels that attach the embryo to the yolk. The eyes may be seen as a bulge on the side of the head. The heart may be located as well as the neural tube that will form the spinal cord. Record the length of the embryo: _____

6. Fertilized eggs may be examined in later development (10, 15, and 20 days) if available. Embryos may be preserved after examination by placing them in vials containing a solution of 70% alcohol.

Drawing Conclusions

1. What is the function of the yolk of the egg?

   _____

   _____

   _____

2. What is the function of the blood vessels from the yolk to the embryo?

   _____

   _____

   _____

3. The functon of the albumen in the egg is to protect the embryo from environmental changes. What structures provide this function in the development of the human embryo?

   _____

   _____

   _____

4. Which body organ is largest at the beginning of development?

   _____

   _____

   _____

Critical Thinking

Ethical Issues of Reproduction

The headlines of newspapers demonstrate the complexity of the ethical issues surrounding the innovations of reproduction. How a person feels about these issues is a result of past experience, religious beliefs, education, and many other factors. There are no right or wrong responses to the following questions. Some examples of the ethical issues of reproduction include:

- *Roe v. Wade* abortion decision being challenged by Supreme Court decision
- surrogate parenting now illegal in several states
- grandmother in South Africa giving birth to her own grandchild (conceived through in vitro fertilization)
- against wishes of relatives, Australian judge ordering frozen embryos to be implanted in surrogate

after millionaire parents killed in plane crash
- daughter becoming pregnant in order to donate aborted fetal tissues to help her father combat Parkinson's disease
- husband suing wife to prevent implantation of frozen embryos after divorce
- selective aborton to choose sex and other genetic characteristics now possible in cases of multiple pregnancies (e.g., twins, triplets, and so forth)
- hundreds of babies born to drug-addicted mothers living in hospitals as boarder babies
- baby with birth defect allowed to die, another with same condition given life-saving surgery; hospital decision based on family's economic ability to care for disabled child
- surgeon providing free surgery to infertile women living on welfare to make conception possible

Examining the Evidence

1. The ethical issues surrounding reproductive function find people on both sides of the dispute. Why do you think that coming to an agreement as to what is "right" or "wrong" in these situations is so difficult?

   _____

   _____

   _____

2. Which interested parties do you think should be on an ethical committee of a hospital or health care agency to determine the course of action in these situations?

   _____

   _____

   _____

3. What factors do you think have most importance in making ethical decisions about these issues (economic, social, religious, legal, etc.)? Give the reasoning that supports your position.

   _____

   _____

   _____

4. List the three issues that concern you the most of those presented earlier or that are now current in the news.

   _____

   _____

   _____

5. Explain your position on one of the three issues you listed in question four.

   _____

   _____

   _____

6. Why might someone have a view that differs from the one you stated in question five?

   _____

   _____

   _____

21 Laboratory Careers

Vapid Vocabulary

Before reading the chapter, review the glossary terms from the chapter in the word search puzzle below. Define each of the terms in the space provided.

```
I  Y  S  Y  N  I  G  S  T  E  D  E  E  R  B  R  N  E  Y  E
M  X  T  Y  S  F  L  N  T  Y  I  F  A  I  S  G  T  A  R  I
M  E  C  I  C  P  E  U  U  R  A  O  Y  Y  T  N  N  R  S  A
U  A  U  Q  R  M  O  N  E  Y  G  R  Y  U  T  P  D  S  R  A
N  X  A  Q  I  E  Q  T  Y  E  N  E  E  O  I  I  I  N  A  L
O  B  A  D  N  R  T  E  U  E  O  N  S  A  G  E  O  E  B  Y
L  Y  E  G  N  T  I  X  G  A  S  S  A  I  G  E  N  N  U  N
O  S  I  Y  G  E  S  I  E  L  I  I  Q  Y  C  R  O  R  G  G
G  D  A  Y  X  I  S  I  G  D  S  C  A  N  G  N  T  T  C  A
Y  Q  T  E  R  A  B  A  A  A  M  E  N  E  E  A  R  Q  A  R
N  A  S  B  G  E  Y  R  E  Y  E  E  Y  A  R  G  N  U  I  S
U  Y  E  U  R  Y  D  C  G  T  A  E  L  S  N  Y  C  E  E
Q  D  O  T  R  Y  N  Y  U  N  A  S  L  A  U  E  T  I  I  U
A  M  T  E  T  R  N  Y  O  T  R  R  M  N  G  N  U  N  Y  A
N  A  M  T  D  A  E  E  S  Y  B  E  T  E  A  E  Y  A  S  Y
A  U  C  Y  S  L  N  R  U  O  I  T  E  I  O  N  D  E  G  A
O  E  E  E  C  I  C  N  X  T  L  N  N  E  E  A  O  T  R  N
Q  U  A  R  A  N  T  I  N  E  A  R  A  G  A  A  O  E  N  N
M  S  R  R  M  E  Q  Y  E  I  C  Q  E  A  S  Q  A  Q  I  N
Y  T  O  U  D  Y  L  O  U  Y  Y  N  Q  R  T  U  E  T  I  E
```

1. Agar- _____

2. Autopsy- _____

3. Calibrate- _____

4. Debris- _____

5. Dexterity- _____

6. Diagnosis- _____

7. Forensic- _____

8. Immunology- _____

9. Quarantine- _____

10. Sediment- _____

Key Search

Find the Key Terms of the chapter by matching the terms to the definitions in the space provided.

Term Tank		
Donor	Microorganism	Phlebotomy
Fomite	Nonpathogen	Recipient
Immunity	Pathogen	Sterile
Infection	Phagocyte	

DEFINITION	KEY TERM
Incision into a vein to withdraw blood	
Free from all living microorganisms	
Microorganism that does not produce disease	
A person who supplies living tissue or who furnishes blood or blood products for transfusion to another person	
Cell that surrounds and destroys microorganisms and foreign particles	
Life form that can be seen only with powerful magnification	
One who receives tissue from another, such as in a blood transfusion	
Microscopic living organism, microbe	
Invasion and multiplication of pathogenic microorganisms in the body tissues	
High level of resistance to certain microorganisms or diseases	
Microorganism that produces disease	

Just the Facts

1. The _ _ Ⓞ _ _ _ _ _ _ _ _ is a medical doctor who examines specimens of body tissue, fluids, and secretions to diagnose disease.

2. Areas of specialization for laboratory technologist include

   _ _ _ _ _ _ _ _ _ _ _ _, chemistry,

   _ _ _ _ _ _ _ _ _ _ _, and immunology.

3. Microbiologists study _ _ _ _ Ⓞ _ _ _, _ _ _ _ _ _,

   _ _ _ _ _ _ _ and other microorganisms that cause disease or may be used to prevent it.

4. Some microorganisms are always present (_ _ _ _ _ _ _ Ⓞ) and some are found temporarily (_ _ _ _ _ _ _ _ _).

5. _ _ _ _ _ _ _ _ _ is a state of disease caused by the presence of pathogenic microorganisms in the body.

6. Four groups of microorganisms that cause disease in humans are _ _ _ _ _ _ _ _ _, fungi, _ _ _ _ _ _ _ _ Ⓞ _ _, and viruses.

7. _ _ _ _ _ _ _ _ _ _ _ _ _ is the study of diseases occurring in human populations.

8. _ _ _ Ⓞ _ _ _ _ _ _ is the study of how the blood cells prevent disease caused by microorganisms.

9. The first line of defense is the _ _ _ Ⓞ, while a second defense is the action of _ _ _ _ _ _ _ _ _ _ _ cells.

10. One of the skills used by the laboratory personnel is the preparation of bacterial cultures using Ⓞ _ _ _ _ _ _ technique.

Use the circled letters to form the answer to this jumble. Clue: What is a bacterial infection that may result from a puncture wound?

_ _ _ _ _ _ _

Concept Applications

Identifying Disease-Causing Microorganisms

Use Table 21-4 in the textbook to label the diagrams of microorganisms in Figure 21-1 A to F. In the spaces provided in Table 21-1, list two diseases that each of these types of organisms cause in humans.

metazoan	fungi	bacteria
rickettsiae	virus	protozoan

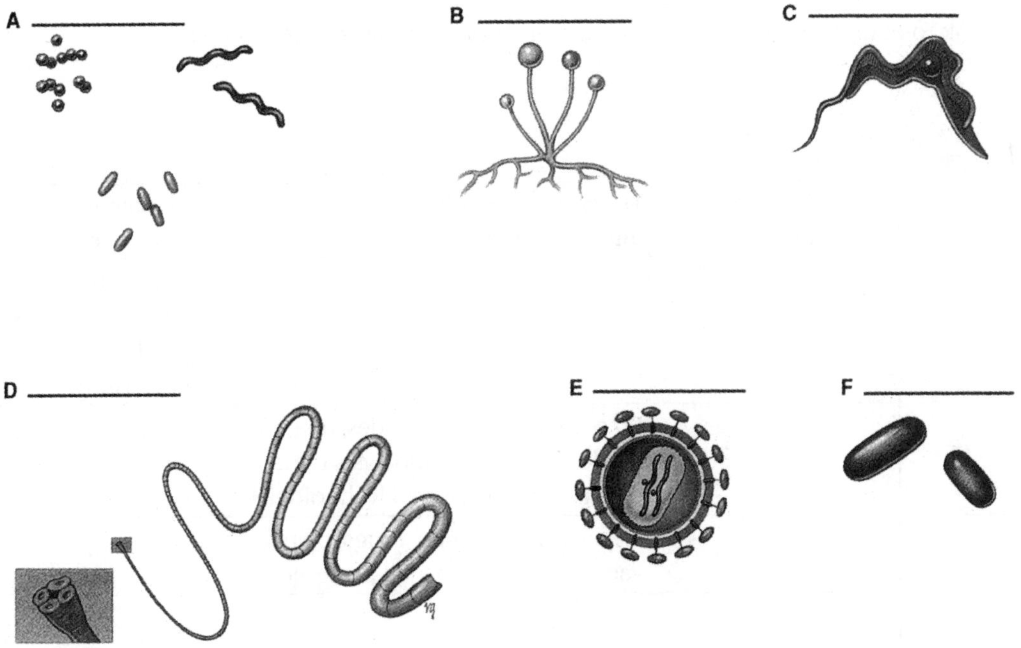

Figure 21-1

TABLE 21-1   Diseases Caused by Microorganism

1. Virus	
2. Bacteria	
3. Yeast	
4. Mold	
5. Metazoan	
6. Protozoan	

Laboratory Careers

Laboratory Skills and Qualities

List three personal qualities and skills that are important in laboratory careers.

1. _____

2. _____

3. _____

Identifying Laboratory Careers

Use the textbook to complete the missing information about laboratory careers in Table 21-2.

TABLE 21-2

Career Title	Years of Education	Description of Job Duties and Opportunities	Credentials Required
			BS, Certified Technologist, some states require licensure
		Preparation of tissue slides, analysis of blood samples, urinalysis under supervision of certified technologist	
		Development of new drugs, plant varieties, environmental protection	
Food scientist			
		Make prostheses including bridges, dentures, crowns, etc	

Applying Your Knowledge

1. The medical doctor who often manages the laboratory and examines body tissues and fluids is called a _____.

2. The _____ would examine urine to assist in diagnosing a bladder infection.

3. The professional who would be involved in the research and study of HIV is probably a _____.

4. The study of body specimens to determine hormonal and chemical changes at the cellular level is performed by a technologist specializing in _____.

5. Safe food processing is evaluated by the _____.

Investigations

Using the Microscope to Identify Microorganisms

Review the directions for use of the microscope found in the textbook in Skill List 21-4. You will be assigned a microorganism or secretion specimen by your teacher. Read all of the directions before beginning this activity. Laboratory activities should be completed only under the supervision of a qualified professional.

Equipment and Supplies

cover slip
eyedropper
microscope
microscope slide
prepared slide of microorganism
unknown specimen
water

Directions

1. Maintain medical asepsis by practicing good handwashing technique.

2. Use the directions for microscope to observe and draw the prepared slide under low, medium, and high power in Figure 21-2.

3. Prepare a wet mount slide by placing a small amount of the unknown specimen in the center of clean slide. Add a drop of water to the specimen if it is not already in a solution.

4. Cover the specimen with a clean cover slip.

5. Use the directions for microscope use to observe and draw the prepared slide under low, medium, and high power in Figure 21-3.

6. Clean and return all materials to the designated location.

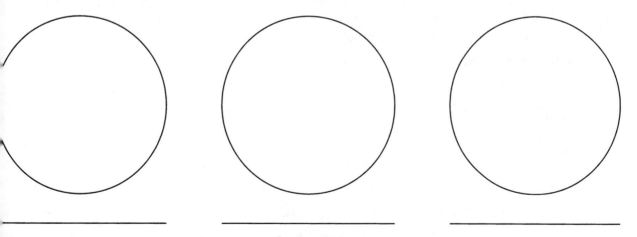

Figure 21-2

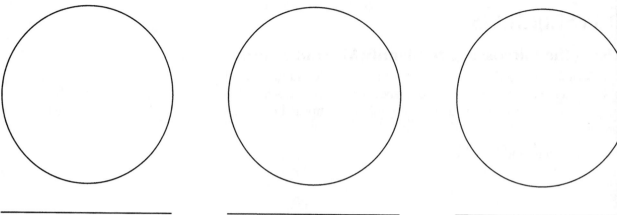

Figure 21-3

Drawing Conclusions

1. How does the "field of vision," or amount of the specimen, compare when the microscope is switched from low to high power?

    _____

    _____

    _____

2. Why is it important to look at the objective from the side when moving it toward the stage?

    _____

    _____

    _____

3. What does *parfocal* mean?

    _____

    _____

    _____

Identifying Microorganisms in the School and Home Environment

Review the information in the textbook regarding preparation of sterile agar plates and transfer of bacteria before beginning this activity. Many bacteria can be found in common household and school environments. Read all of the directions before beginning this activity. Laboratory activities should be completed only under the supervision of a qualified professional.

Equipment and Supplies

autoclave or bleach
grease pencil or china marker
incubator
sterile culture swab
sterile nutrient agar plate

Directions

1. Maintain medical asepsis by practicing good handwashing technique.

2. Prepare a sterile agar plate and culture swab. A wooden cotton swab can be sterilized for use as a culture swab.

3. Collect a specimen by rubbing the cotton swab on a surface in your environment. Do not allow the cotton swab to touch any other surface.

4. Open the sterile plate to inoculate the agar with the culture swab. Close the plate immediately.

5. Discard the culture swab in the proper receptacle.

6. Mark the bottom of a sterile agar plate with the site of specimen collection, date, and your initials.

7. Place the closed plate in an incubator at 37° C. Place the plate upside down to prevent condensation or liquid from forming on the specimen.

8. Incubate the plate for 3 or 4 days. Make observations for each 24-hour period.

9. Count the number of different types of bacterial colonies on the plate. Record your results.

10. Compare your results with other locations in the environment.

11. To prevent the spread of unknown microorganisms, sterilize or disinfect the agar before discarding it.

12. You may repeat the procedure by testing only for airborne microorganisms. The plate should be exposed to the air in different locations for a designated length of time before incubation for this activity.

13. Clean and return all materials to the designated location.

Drawing Conclusions

1. How many and what type of colonies of bacteria did your plate show after incubation?

_____

_____

_____

2. In what area of the environment did your class find the most bacterial growth?

_____

_____

_____

3. Why is it important to sterilize or disinfect the culture plates before discarding them?

_____

_____

_____

4. Why is 37° C used for incubation of the microorganisms?

_____

_____

_____

5. Why weren't the bacteria visible before incubation?

_____

_____

_____

Demonstrating the Effect of Antibiotics on Bacteria

Antibiotics are chemical substances that kill microorganisms or inhibit their growth. Most antibiotics are made from natural waste products of fungi and bacteria. Antibiotics have varied levels of effectiveness in killing different bacteria. Before prescribing an antibiotic, it is helpful to know which one would be most effective. The following activity will determine which antibiotic is most effective in inhibiting the growth of a known bacteria.

Antibiotic-resistant types of bacteria are common in hospitals, because so many antibiotics are used in those facilities.

Review the information in the textbook about the correct way to transfer bacteria before beginning this activity. Nonpathogenic bacteria and antibiotic dots may be purchased for this activity from a biological supply service.

Read all of the directions before beginning this activity. Laboratory activities should be completed only under the supervision of a qualified professional.

Equipment and Supplies

antibiotic disks
autoclave or bleach
china marker
incubator
known nonpathogenic bacteria
sterile culture swab or inoculating loop
sterile forceps or antibiotic disk dispenser
sterile nutrient agar plate

Directions

1. Maintain medical asepsis by practicing good handwashing technique.

2. Use sterile technique to transfer the known nonpathogenic bacteria from the culture tube to a sterile nutrient agar plate. Streak the surface evenly without breaking the surface of the agar.

3. Use a sterile forceps or antibiotic dispenser to space three or four different antibiotic dots evenly on the surface of the agar.

4. Use a china maker to label each section of the agar plate on the bottom of the agar plate to indicate the date, your initials, and the types of antibiotics used.

5. Place the Petri dish upside down in an incubator at 37° C for 3 or 4 days.

6. Observe the agar plate for clear areas around each antibiotic disk. The halo, or "zone of inhibition," indicates that the antibiotic inhibited the growth of the bacteria in that area. The size of the zone indicates how effective the antibiotic is in stopping the bacterial growth.

7. Measure the width of each zone of inhibition. Record the results in Table 21-3.

8. Sterilize or disinfect the cultures before discarding them.

9. Clean and return all materials to the designated location.

TABLE 21-3   **Antibiotic Effects Results**

Type of microorganism:	
Type of antibiotic	Size of halo
Type of antibiotic	Size of halo
Type of antibiotic	Size of halo
Type of antibiotic	Size of halo

Drawing Conclusions

1. Which antibiotic was most effective against the bacteria?

   _____

   _____

   _____

2. What are four items necessary for the growth of bacterial colonies?

   _____

   _____

   _____

3. What are two precautions that you used during the activity to protect yourself and the agar medium from contamination with unknown microorganisms?

   _____

   _____

   _____

4. What are two potential sources of error in your activity?

   _____

   _____

   _____

Demonstrating the Effect of Disinfectants on Bacteria

Review the information in the textbook about the correct method to transfer bacteria before beginning this activity. Disinfectants are chemical compounds that inhibit the growth of microorganisms. Non-pathogenic bacteria may be purchased for this activity from a biological supply service.

Read all of the directions before beginning this activity. Laboratory activities should be completed only under the supervision of a qualified professional.

Equipment and Supplies

autoclave or bleach
disinfectants
incubator
nonpathogenic bacteria
sterile forceps
sterile nutrient agar plate
sterile swab or inoculating loop
sterile filter disks soaked with disinfectants

Directions

1. Maintain medical asepsis by practicing good handwashing technique.

2. Transfer the known nonpathogenic bacteria from the culture tube to a sterile agar plate. Streak the agar evenly without breaking the surface.

3. Dip a small sterile filter disk into a household disinfectant.

4. Use sterile forceps to space three or four different disinfectant filter dots evenly on the surface of the agar.

5. Use a china marker to label each section on the bottom of the agar plate to indicate the date, your initials, and the types of disinfectants used.

6. Place the Petri dish upside down in an incubator at 37° C for 3 or 4 days.

7. Observe the agar plate for clear areas around each disinfectant disk. The halo, or "zone of inhibition," indicates that the disinfectant inhibited the growth of the bacteria in that area. The size of the halo indicates the effectiveness of the disinfectant in stopping bacterial growth.

8. Measure the width of each zone of inhibition. Record the results in Table 21-4.

9. Sterilize or disinfect the cultures before discarding them.

10. Clean and return all materials to the designated location.

TABLE 21-4   Disinfectant Effects Results

Type of microorganism:	
Type of disinfectant	Size of halo
Type of disinfectant	Size of halo
Type of disinfectant	Size of halo
Type of disinfectant	Size of halo

Drawing Conclusions

1. Which disinfectant was most effective against the bacteria?

_____

_____

_____

2. What are two precautions that you used during the activity to protect yourself and the agar medium from contamination with unknown microorganisms?

_____

_____

_____

3. What are two sources of error in your activity?

_____

_____

_____

4. What is the difference between a disinfectant and an antibiotic?

_____

_____

_____

Critical Thinking

Laboratory Safety

No set of policies and procedures can cover all of the situations in which hazards in the medical laboratory might occur. However, practicing some simple rules and using common sense can make the laboratory a safe environment. The following are some of the rules of safety that apply to any laboratory environment.

Laboratory Safety Guidelines

1 Read all instructions about any unfamiliar procedure before attempting it.
2 Do not eat, drink, smoke, or chew gum in the laboratory area. Do not place supplies, equipment, or chemicals in the mouth.
3 Keep the laboratory area clean and free from debris. Store equipment and supplies in the designated manner and location after use.
4 Wear gloves when handling body secretions and at all times if open sores or cuts are present on the hands. Wash hands frequently and when any laboratory chemical or specimen is accidentally touched.
5 Handle all laboratory equipment with care and follow the manufacturer's instructions at all times. Report damaged equipment and supplies promptly. Clean any spills or breakage promptly and in an appropriate manner.
6 Do not replace used chemicals into stock bottles. Handle chemicals, test tubes, and other supplies and equipment with the appropriate utensil. Wear safety glasses and masks as needed when handling toxic chemicals and when running the autoclave.

7 Do not wear jewelry or clothing that hangs loose or dangles. Contain hair in a band or net to keep it away from the face and neck. Wear a standard laboratory jacket and closed-toed shoes.

8 Avoid horseplay and other dangerous behaviors at all times. Report any accident or injury to the supervisor immediately.

9 Keep visitors and nonlaboratory personnel in a designated area away from the laboratory work.

10 Know the location of and how to use diagnostic and laboratory equipment, including a fire extinguisher, fire blanket, and laboratory shower.

Examining the Evidence

1. What does the phrase "common sense" mean?

_____

_____

_____

2. Give an explanation of the importance of each of the 10 safety guidelines.

1. _____

_____

_____

2. _____

_____

_____

3. _____

_____

_____

4. _____

_____

_____

5. _____

_____

_____

6. _____

_____

_____

7. _____

_____

_____

8. _____

_____

_____

9. _____

_____

_____

10. _____

_____

_____

3. For what other reason, in addition to safety, would it be important to follow the guidelines?

_____

_____

_____

4. Which individual in the laboratory is most responsible for laboratory safety?

_____

_____

_____

22 Imaging Careers

Vapid Vocabulary

Before reading the chapter, review the glossary terms from the chapter in the word search puzzle below. Define each of the terms in the space provided.

```
N O I T N E V R E T N I Z O N G G D R C
I O D Y D A P M M P A A O M D R N I T C
E U I A V R D O M A I R O T E E I O T M
N I M Y O V A E T Y M O T S U R G A T I
Y N I V I G O T M O A M O Y U N A M V M
M Z D I D Y O O Y U S N O A M N M N Y M
I E I V R E V G E R A I O G E T I Y T S
T M Y M R V E N M N T P O I R T A A P E
U A A O N A T M C Y A E M I T A V A I N
N T P T I M I E I Q G T I M D O P N A S
I I I I O Y N M U N Y T A I O A T H I I
Y N O L R I V E N A O T M N Z Z R M Y T
R A A M I A V U V M P I Y Q Y M T R N I
G T I M T T Y I E M A M T Y O A I V E Z
D R A T T T Y D V A O M N A A N O Z M E
I P T R R T I O G A I M V T I G M V U Z
A I D I G A D A M D U I U M N D O I O M
T I C N C I E I R O O E M E Z N A M N O
C O O I N O P P M I N O O E N A O R D T
C A M R A N E O N T T T A E U Z T M D I
```

1. Imaging- _____

2. Intervention- _____

3. Mammography- _____

4. Media- _____

5. Opaque- _____

6. Radiation- _____

7. Radioisotope- _____

8. Resonance- _____

9. Sensitize- _____

10. Utility- _____

Key Search

Find the Key Terms of the chapter by matching the terms to the definitions in the space provided.

Term Tank		
Echocardiography	Radiographic contrast media	
Fluoroscopy	Radiography	
Isotope	Tomography	
Polarity	Ultrasound	

DEFINITION	KEY TERM
Chemical that does not permit passage of x-rays	
Visualization of deep structures of the body by recording reflections of sound waves directed into the tissues	
Recording the position and motion of the heart walls or its internal structures using ultrasonic waves	
Making film records of internal structures by passing radiographs or gamma rays through the body to make images on specially sensitized film	
Immediate visualization of part of the body on a screen using radiography	
One or more forms of an atom with a difference in the number of neutrons	
Radiograph producing a detained cross-section of tissue at a predetermined depth	
Distinction between positive and negative charges of particles	

Just the Facts

1. Radiology technologists work under the direction of a Ⓞ _ _ _ _ _ _ _ _ and may specialize in one area of diagnosis or treatment.

2. Radiology work has some hazard of radiation exposure, so each worker wears a _ _ _ _ _ _ _ _ _ that records the level of exposure to radiologic materials.

3. Radioactive compounds may be _ _ _ _ _ Ⓞ _ _ into the bloodstream, _ _ _ _ _ Ⓞ _ _ _, or _ _ _ _ _ _ _ _.

4. _ _ _ _ _ _ _ _ _ _ _ _ _ _ _ _ _ _ _ technicians may work in the radiology department and monitor or test the action of the heart.

5. _ Ⓞ _ technologists measure the electrical activity of the brain.

6. The field of radiography has expanded greatly as modern methods of imaging have combined the use of _ _ _ _ _ _ _ _ _ with radiographic procedures.

7. _ _ _ _ _ Ⓞ _ _ _ _ _ _ _ _ _ _ _ tomography uses computers and radiographic technique to visualize the metabolic activities of the body as well as its structure.

8. _ _ _ _ _ _ Ⓞ _ _ _ _ _ _ _ _ _ _ imaging is a process that creates superb image resolution and tissue contrast.

9. A _ Ⓞ _ _ _ _ _ _ _ is a radiograph of the breast used to detect cancer.

10. Near infrared _ _ _ _ _ _ _ _ _ _ _ _ Ⓞ is a technique that allows _ _ _ _ _ _ _ _ _ _ _ measuring of cerebral functions.

Use the circled letters to form the answer to this jumble. Clue: What is the property of cells that allows radiologists to use magnets to produce images?

_ _ _ _ _ _ _ _

Concept Applications

Imaging Careers

Imaging Skills and Qualities

List three personal qualities and skills that are important in imaging careers.

1. _____

2. _____

3. _____

Identifying Imaging Careers

Use the textbook to complete the missing information about imaging careers in Table 22-1.

TABLE 22-1

Career Title	Years of Education	Description of Job Duties and Opportunities	Credentials Required
		Produce two-dimensional images of internal organs using sound waves at high frequency	
		Transfer and position the client, select materials for making images including radiopaque	
		Use computers and magnets to produce an image of the internal soft tissues	
		Prepare and administer radioactive compounds	
	On the job or 1- to 2-year program		

Applying Your Knowledge

1. The imaging health care worker who might be found in the emergency department to assist with diagnosis of a broken arm would be the _____.

2. An _____ performs tests that may help to determine fetal age.

3. A brain tumor might be diagnosed using the radioactive tests performed by the

   _____.

4. The health care worker who may assist with diagnosing abnormal electrical activity of the brain is the _____.

5. The _____ would administer the radiation treatment for many types of cancer.

Investigations

Determining the Effect of Light Rays

Light and radiograph waves come from the same electromagnetic spectrum and share many of the same properties. Work in groups of two to three people for this activity. Read all of the directions before beginning this activity. Laboratory activities should be completed only under the supervision of a qualified professional.

Equipment and Supplies

construction paper (optional)
flashlight
penlight
yardstick

Directions

1. Hold a flashlight perpendicular to the wall at a distance of 1 foot.

2. Measure the diameter of the image produced by the beam on the wall.

3. Repeat the procedure when the flashlight is held 2, 3, 4, and 5 feet from the wall. Record the results in Table 22-2.

4. Repeat steps 1 to 3 using the penlight as the energy source. Record the results in Table 22-2.

5. Using the flashlight as the energy source, repeat steps 1 to 3 while holding a piece of construction paper 6 inches from the wall between the wall and beam of the flashlight during all measurements. Record the results in Table 22-2.

TABLE 22-2   Diameter of Light Beam

Distance	1 foot	2 feet	3 feet	4 feet	5 feet
Flashlight					
Penlight					
Construction paper					

Drawing Conclusions

1. How does the area covered by the beam from the light source that is near the wall compare with the area covered at a greater distance?

   _____

   _____

   _____

2. Was the beam produced by the light source stronger or weaker in intensity as it was moved farther from the wall?

_____

_____

_____

3. Why does the operator of radiographic equipment maintain as great a distance from the beam as possible?

_____

_____

_____

4. How does the construction paper placed between the light source and wall represent the action of a lead shield used in radiography?

_____

_____

_____

Critical Thinking

Calculating the Intensity of Energy Sources

Beams of energy follow the law of intensity called the *inverse square law of radiation*. It states that the intensity of the radiation beam is inversely proportional to the square of the distance from the source.

Examining the Evidence

1. Use Table 22-2 to calculate the "intensity" of light produced by the flashlight from the distances measured. What are these values?

_____

_____

_____

2. Does the inverse square law apply to the beam produced by the light source?

_____

_____

_____

23 Nursing Careers

Vapid Vocabulary

Before reading the chapter, review the glossary terms from the chapter in the word search puzzle below. Define each of the terms in the space provided.

```
T S E G N I L X M R I P T R R A A P R T
E R L M E I E A E R R L D P L D I E A P
P I C R E P O C N E I T I T T E A T A L
C E E R A R E I J I R N R P L U G P C R
N E R T H P L U L I R P D I T R O L I U
A R N I T U D E G O U U D I D E R N R A
I A S A O I O N O E G R U L T U R T I C
E N C P C D R I I N I E P N Y R O G M O
L L T E I N I E L E I D E E I I D S P L
E E C R I L D C O I D E R S U T N A C E
U E L L A U R U E G M R I U A A T A E I
R U M G D V A I E Y D L P D L N R I U E
T P D R D U E H E H O A H M R S L T D I
E L E R T E R N I Y R M E L C A L A E D
T O D P T P D D O T E I R E D R R T R E
T S I I O E R D I U J T A A O D A R I A
N J C M R I L L T A S P L C A R N O P U
R U E I C D O R L U L O U E V D U P U I
D E E E Y T L G C E L U E D I E P E E I
P D E T E E D E E S I U P D R E A E O I
```

1. Apex- _____

2. Hygiene- _____

3. Ingest- _____

4. Intravenous- _____

5. Optimal- _____

6. Periodic- _____

7. Peripheral- _____

8. Prejudice- _____

9. Receptacle- _____

10. Urinal- _____

Key Search

Find the Key Terms of the chapter by matching the terms to the definitions in the space provided.

Term Tank		
Apical	Perinatal	
Asepsis	Pulse	
Emesis	Unit	
Intravenous	Vital	

DEFINITION	**KEY TERM**
Part of a facility, including equipment and supplies, organized to provide specific care	
Necessary to life	
Heartbeat that can be felt, or palpated, on surface arteries as the artery walls expand	
Pertaining to the period shortly before and after birth	
Process of removing pathogenic microorganisms or protecting against infection by such organisms	
Within a vein or veins	
Pertaining to, or located at, the apex of the heart	
Vomit	

Just the Facts

1. _ _ _ _ _ Ⓞ make up the largest group of health care workers, with more than 2 million jobs.

2. The function of the nurse is to promote _ _ _ _ _ _ _ health and _ _ _ _ _ Ⓞ _ care during illness.

3. Three levels of nursing care include the _ _ _ _ _ _ _ _ _ _ _ nurse, _ Ⓞ _ _ _ _ _ _ _ _ _ _ _ _ _ _ _ _ _ nurse, and nurse _ _ _ _ _ _ _ _ _.

4. Advanced preparation by the registered nurse may lead to work as a nurse _ _ _ _ _ _ _ _ _ _ _ _ _, clinical nurse _ _ _ _ _ _ _ _ _ _, nurse _ _ _ _ _ _ _ _ _ _ _ _ _, or nurse _ _ _ _ _ Ⓞ _.

5. Areas of specialization for the _ Ⓞ _ _ _ _ _ _ _ _ nurse include units, such as the operating room, recovery room, critical care, and emergency department.

6. Nurse assistants may provide care in the patient's home and are called _ _ _ _ Ⓞ _ _ _ assistants.

7. Within a 24-hour period, the fluid that is taken into the body and eliminated from the body should be approximately equal in volume to maintain the balance of the _ _ _ _ _ _ _ _ _ _ _ _ _ _ and Ⓞ _ _ _ _ needed to perform body processes.

8. Oral intake is considered to be anything that is _ _ _ Ⓞ _ _ at room temperature and taken by _ _ _ _ _.

9. Ⓞ _ _ _ _ _ _ _ _ _ _ _ _ _ exercises are designed to move the muscles and tendons of the joints for patients that are not able to move independently or have limited abilities.

10. Maintaining an orderly and safe environment for care of the patient is the responsibility of _ Ⓞ _ health care _ _ _ _ _ _ _ _ _ Ⓞ _ _ _ _.

Use the circled letters to form the answer to this jumble. Clue: What is the phrase used when the patient is offered at least 100 mL of liquid every hour?

_ _ _ _ _ _   _ _ _ _ _ _

Concept Applications

Recording Daily Care

Review the information provided in Chapter 2 and Chapter 6 for Therapeutic and Diagnostic Careers regarding assessment and recording of vital signs.

Use the information provided in Figure 23-1, Mrs. Jewel's hospital stay graphic sheet, to complete the care flow sheet in Figure 23-2.

Drawing Conclusions

1. How well dis Mrs. Jewel eat breakfast and lunch on the day recorded?

   _____

   _____

   _____

2. Why is the dinner meal omitted by the health care assistant?

   _____

   _____

   _____

3. What is the level of responsiveness and orientation of Mrs. Jewel?

   _____

   _____

   _____

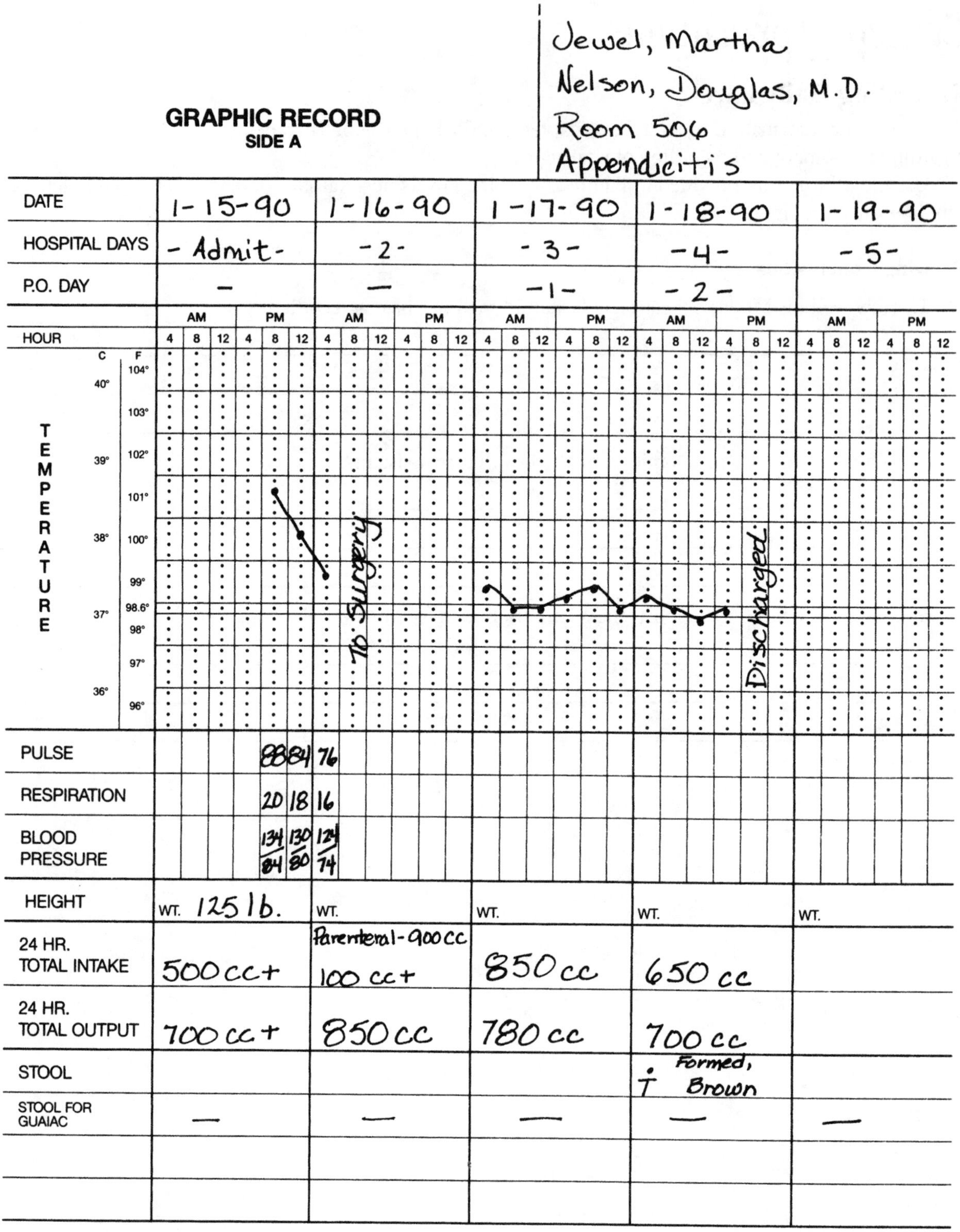

GRAPHIC RECORD
SIDE A

Jewel, Martha
Nelson, Douglas, M.D.
Room 506
Appendicitis

DATE	1-15-90						1-16-90						1-17-90						1-18-90						1-19-90					
HOSPITAL DAYS	-Admit-						-2-						-3-						-4-						-5-					
P.O. DAY	—						—						-1-						-2-											

Temperature graph (Temperature 96°–104° F / 36°–40° C). Notations on graph: "To Surgery" (1-16-90), temperature plot across 1-17-90 to 1-18-90 near 98.6°, "Discharged" (1-19-90).

	AM	PM	AM	PM	AM	PM	AM	PM	AM	PM
PULSE		88 84 76								
RESPIRATION		20 18 16								
BLOOD PRESSURE		134/84 130/80 124/74								

HEIGHT	WT. 125 lb.	WT.	WT.	WT.	WT.
24 HR. TOTAL INTAKE	500 cc+	Parenteral-900 cc 100 cc+	850 cc	650 cc	
24 HR. TOTAL OUTPUT	700 cc+	850 cc	780 cc	700 cc	
STOOL				Formed, ↑ Brown	
STOOL FOR GUAIAC	—	—	—	—	—

Figure 23-1 *Graphic record*

CARE FLOW SHEET

CLIENT NAME: _Jewel, Martha_ ____   ROOM NO.: _506_ ____

	7-3	3-11	11-7
Bath/Shower/Bedbath	Shower 9:00 SS		
Hair Care	9:15 SS		
Back Rub/Skin Care	9:15 SS		
Nails	—		
Shave	—		
Oral Hygiene	Self 8:00 SS		
Temperature			
Pulse			
Respiration			
Blood Pressure			
Urine Output			
Bowel Movement			
Level of Consciousness	Alert SS		
Orientation	Oriented x3 SS		
Breakfast (% Eaten)	80%		
Lunch (% Eaten)	50%		
Dinner (% Eaten)	—		
Clinitest	—		
Acetest	—		
Sleep/Rest	—		
Specimen	—		
Other	—		

SIGNATURE: _SSmith_ ____   TITLE: _LPN_ ____   DATE: _1-18-90_ ____

SIGNATURE: _____   TITLE: _____   DATE: _____

SIGNATURE: _____   TITLE: _____   DATE: _____

Figure 23-2 *Care flow sheet*

Assessing Tissue Integrity and Safety Needs

Study the following tissue integrity survey in Figure 23-3 and the safety assessment in Figure 23-4 for Mrs. Jewel during her hospital stay.

Jewel, Martha
Nelson, Douglas, M.D.
Room 506
Appendicitis

ASSESSMENT FORM
- TISSUE INTEGRITY
- PATIENT SAFETY

TISSUE INTEGRITY ASSESSMENT FORM

Identify any patient at risk of developing pressure sores. Assess the seven clinical condition parameters to determine a patient risk score. Patients with a score of twelve or more should be considered at risk of developing pressure sores. Initiate preventive protocol per patient care plan.

CLINICAL CONDITION PARAMETERS	adm.	72hrs.	1wk.
GENERAL PHYSICAL CONDITION (health problems) Good (minor) .... 0 Fair (acute/chronic - but stable) .... 1 Poor (acute/chronic - not stable) .... 2 Terminal 3	0	0	
LEVEL OF CONSCIOUSNESS (to commands) Alert (responds readily) .... 0 Lethargic (slow to respond) .... 1 Semi-comatose or Confused .... 2 (responds only to painful/verbal stimuli) Comatose (no response to stimuli) 3	0	0	
ACTIVITY Ambulatory without assistance .... 0 Ambulatory with assistance .... 2 Chair and/or bed only .... 4 Confined to bed 6	2	2	
MOBILITY - RANGE OF MOTION Full active range of motion .... 0 Moves with limited assistance .... 2 Moves only with assistance .... 4 Immobile 6	2	2	
GENERAL SKIN CONDITION Healthy (clean, clear, supple) .... 0 Fair (rashes or abrasions) .... 2 Poor (dry, poor tugor, advanced age) .... 6 Edema, reddened areas, "thin skin" .... 8 Pressure sore (document on Flowsheet) ... 12	0	0	
INCONTINENCE (bowel and/or bladder) None .... 0 Foley catheter .... 1 Occasional (<3 per 24hr) .... 2 Usually (>3 per 24hr) .... 4 Total (no control) 6	0	0	
NUTRITION (for age and size) Good (eats/drinks 75-100% of meals) .... 0 Fair (eats/drinks 50-75% of meals) .... 1 Tube Feeding/Hyperalimentation .... 2 Poor (unable or refuses to eat or drink) 3	1	0	
TOTAL SCORE	5	4	

	Date	Init.	Signature
Adm.	1-15-90	SS	S. Smith, LPN
72hrs.	1-17-90	SS	S. Smith, LPN
1wk.			

Figure 23-3 *Assessment form*

Jewel, Martha
Nelson, Douglas, M.D.
Room 506
Appendicitis

PATIENT SAFETY ASSESSMENT FORM

Identify any patient at risk for fall by assessing the 11 parameters listed and assigning a score (0=least risk and 5=greatest risk). Patients with a score of 15 or above should be considered at risk for a fall and a care plan with appropriate nursing intervention should be developed.

CLINICAL PARAMETERS		adm.	72hrs.	1wk.
1. Unsteady on feet		2	4	
2. Poor eyesight (glasses=1)		1	1	
3. Changes in environment		1	3	
4. Drugs or alcohol		0	0	
5. Physical disabilities		0	0	
6. Multiple diagnosis		0	0	
7. Language barrier		0	0	
8. Neurological problems		0	0	
9. Attitude		1	2	
10. Confused & disoriented	15pts.	0	0	
11. Previous fall	15pts.	0	0	
TOTAL SCORE		4	10	

	Date	Init.	Signature
Adm.	1-15-90	S.S.	S. Smith LPN
72hrs.	1-17-90	S.S.	S. Smith LPN
1wk.			

Figure 23-4 *Patient safety assessment form*

Drawing Conclusions

1. How did the safety assessment change during the first 72 hours of Mrs. Jewel's stay in the hospital?

_____

_____

_____

2. What might have caused the change in the risk factors considered in this assessment?

_____

_____

_____

Temperature Conversion and Charting Vital Signs

Convert the following temperature readings and use the information to chart the following vital signs in Figure 23-5.

DATE	TIME	VITAL SIGNS			
9/1	8:00 A.M.	BP 124/98	P 76	R 20	T 98.6° F orally
	12:00 P.M.	BP 122/76	P 78	R 16	T 98.2° F orally
	4:00 P.M.	BP 120/82	P 70	R 18	T 99.0° F orally
	8:00 P.M.	BP 118/76	P 64	R 22	T 102.0° F rectally
9/2	12:00 A.M.	BP 124/78	P 80	R 26	T 104.2° F rectally
	8:00 A.M.	BP 116/76	P 68	R 16	T 98.2° F orally
	4:00 P.M.	BP 122/82	P 72	R 20	T 98.6° F orally
9/3	8:00 A.M.	BP 120/76	P 68	R 16	T 98.2° F orally
	4:00 P.M.	BP 126/98	P 74	R 14	T 98.6° F orally

GRAPHIC RECORD

UR	2400	0400	0800	1200	1600	2000	2400	0400	0800	1200	1600	2000	2400	0400	0800	1200	1600	2000	2400	0400	0800	1200	1600	2000
2.																								
1.5																								
1.																								
0.5																								
0.																								
9.5																								
9.																								
8.5																								
8.																								
7.5																								
7.																								
6.5																								
6.																								

PULSE

ATION

TIME				
2400				
0400				
0800				
1200				
1600				
2000				

Figure 23-5 *Graphic record*

Graphing Vital Signs

Using the information provided in Figure 23-6 to chart the vital signs, fluid balance, and care record for Ms. Betternow.

DATE   TIME   OBSERVATIONS
10/1   3:30 P.M.   Admitted to hospital, weight 134 pounds, height 5'4".

Admission assessment includes notice of cast on right arm, skin pale with perspiration, c/o poor appetite due to inability to hold utensils and prepare food with left arm only, dressing on right thigh dry with some old serosanguineous stains, 3 cm × 5 cm in size, arrived walking with some limp in left leg, alert and states she does not feel well, has pain in the left leg, states she was in an automobile accident 3 days previously, abdominal sounds heard frequently, abdomen flat and soft when palpated, breath sounds clear and dry, states she has not had a bowel movement for 2 days, darkened and raised area noted on right forehead. Safety and intake and output procedures explained per doctor's orders. Vitals BP 132/86, P 104, R 24, T 100.0° F orally.

    10/1   5:00 P.M.   Urine output 500 cc clear yellow. Dinner intake complete meal including 1 carton of milk, 1 glass of juice, 1 serving mashed potatoes with 1 slice roast beef, 1 serving of gelatin, 1 serving green beans, states she feels better after eating.

    10/1   8:00 P.M.   Vitals BP 140/90, P 100, R 20, T 99.6° F orally. Urine output 350 cc clear yellow. 200 cc water missing from water pitcher. 1 cup ice cubes and 1 soda consumed since dinner.

    10/2   8:00 A.M.   Vitals BP 144/92, P 102, R 22, T 102.2° F orally. c/o HA. LOC somewhat lethargic. 200 cc urine output, dark yellow. Breakfast and a.m. care refused. Doctor called, NPO order given.

    10/2   10:00 A.M.   200 cc dark yellow urine output. LOC lethargic, disoriented ×3. Daily care including bedbath, backrub, and linen change given. c/o distention. Vitals BP 146/94, P 106, R 26, T 100.2° F.

    10/2   11:00 A.M.   Transfer to surgery.

    10/3   5:00 P.M.   Return from surgery. Assessment including shallow breath sounds, LOC lethargic, oriented, bandage on head (turban) dry without spots. Vitals BP 126/78, P 80, R 14, T 94.4° F. Urinary catheter in place, output 200 cc dark yellow urine, IV in place right forearm, insertion site dry and intact.

    10/3   8:00 P.M.   LOC alert, oriented. Ice chips ×3 glasses consumed since 5:00 P.M., 1 cup juice consumed. Urine output 200 cc light yellow. IV site dry and intact.

    10/4   12:00 A.M.   Vitals BP 120/76, P 78, R 16, T 98.6° F. Intake 1 soda, 1 glass juice. Urine output 300 cc, yellow. IV site dry and intact.

    10/4   4:00 A.M.   Vitals BP 126/78, P 80, R 18, T 98.8° F. IV site intact.

    10/4   8:00 A.M.   Vitals BP 120/78, P 76, R 16, T 98.0° F. IV DC'd per MD order by RN. Breakfast consumed including 1 glass juice, 1 cup decaffeinated coffee, 1 slice toast, 1 cup oatmeal, 2 cups water. LOC alert, oriented. Urine output 400 cc clear, yellow. Catheter removed by LPN per MD order. Bedbath, backrub, linen change, and A.M. care given.

    10/4   12:00 P.M.   Vitals BP 124/74, P 74, R 16, T 98.4° F. Urine output 200 cc clear yellow. Bowel movement ×1, formed brown moderate amount of stool.

    10/4   4:00 P.M.   Vitals BP 118/74, P 70, R 16, T 98.0° F. Urine output 250 cc clear yellow.

    10/4   8:00 P.M.   Vitals BP 116/76, P 68, R 14, T 98.4° F. Urine output 350 cc clear yellow.

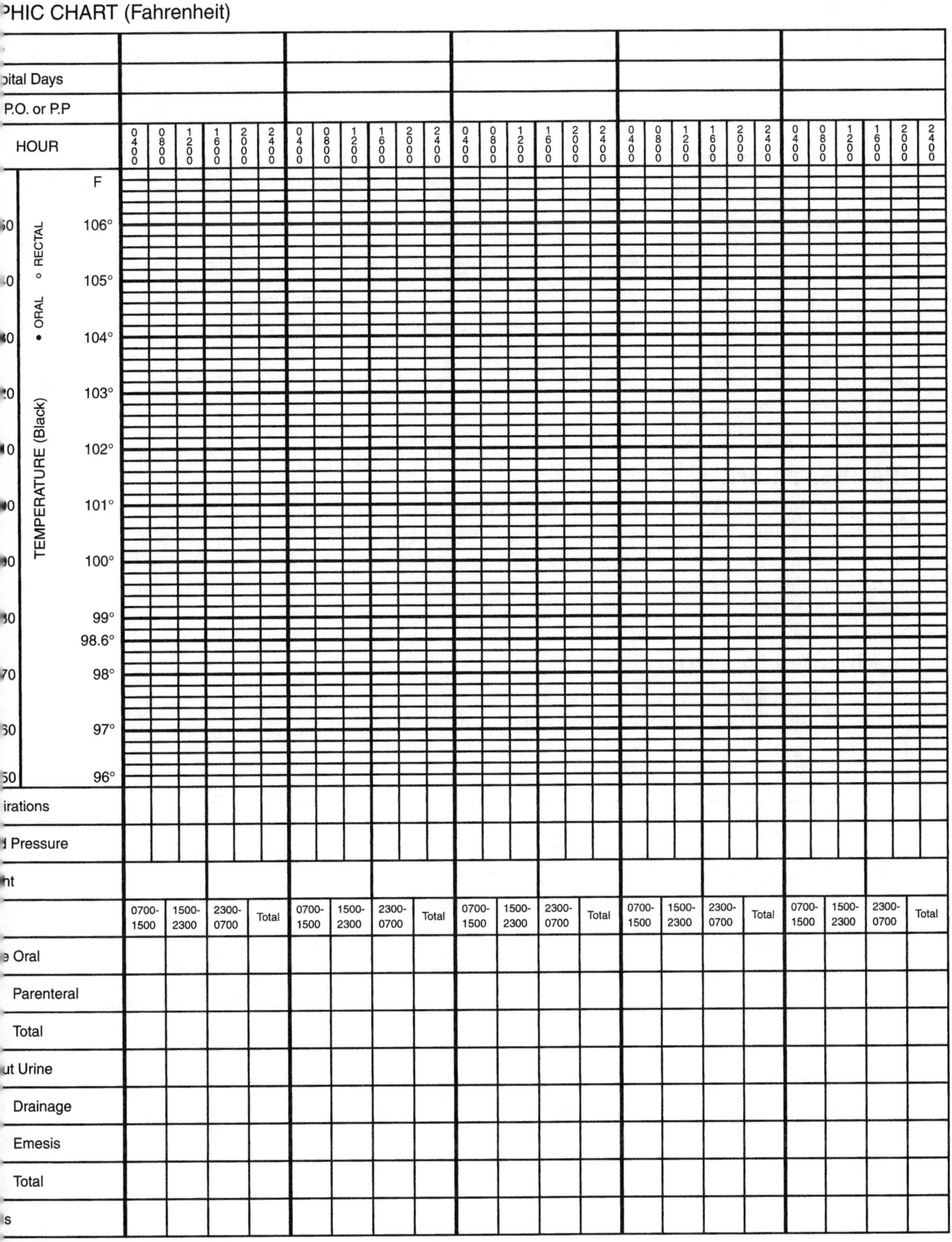

PHIC CHART (Fahrenheit)

pital Days

P.O. or P.P

HOUR	0400	0800	1200	1600	2000	2400	0400	0800	1200	1600	2000	2400	0400	0800	1200	1600	2000	2400	0400	0800	1200	1600	2000	2400	0400	0800	1200	1600	2000	2400

TEMPERATURE (Black)

• ORAL   ○ RECTAL

F
106°
105°
104°
103°
102°
101°
100°
99°
98.6°
98°
97°
96°

irations

Pressure

ht

	0700-1500	1500-2300	2300-0700	Total	0700-1500	1500-2300	2300-0700	Total	0700-1500	1500-2300	2300-0700	Total	0700-1500	1500-2300	2300-0700	Total	0700-1500	1500-2300	2300-0700	Total
e Oral																				
Parenteral																				
Total																				
ut Urine																				
Drainage																				
Emesis																				
Total																				

Figure 23-6 *Graphic chart*

Drawing Conclusions

1. Why was Ms. Betternow made NPO by her physician?

   _____

   _____

   _____

2. What is one explanation for the deterioration (decline) in Ms. Betternow's level of responsiveness?

   _____

   _____

   _____

3. What is the health care assistant's responsibility concerning dressings and intravenous sites?

   _____

   _____

   _____

Reading a Kardex

The Kardex is a card file used in health care that contains information taken from the record or chart for daily care. It is a summary of the care that is ordered. The Kardex is a quick and easy reference and is completed in pencil so that the information may be updated as needed. Figure 23-7A and B represent a sample Kardex for a hospitalized client. In the space provided, organize the tasks to be completed during the day shift.

Applying Your Knowledge

1. Why would it or would it not be more efficient to organize the tasks for more than one client by the type of task or by the time by which each task must be completed?

   _____

   _____

   _____

2. What is the diagnosis for this client?

   _____

   _____

   _____

3. Why would it or would it not be acceptable for this client to walk to a day room and buy a snack?

   _____

   _____

   _____

MODE OF ADMISSION: ED ☐   DIRECT ADMIT ☒   TRANSFER ☐

DATE	VITAL SIGN FREQUENCY	DATE	PERSONAL - ORAL HYGIENE	DATE	TREATMENTS	DATE	SPECIAL INSTRUCTIONS
5/30	T.P.R.: QID		COMPLETE:	5/30	Clinitest & Acetest 1/2hr ac & hs		
5/30	B.P.: QID		SELF WITH HELP:				
	NEURO CHECKS:		SELF CARE:				
			PERICARE:				
5/30	DAILY WT.:						
			REHABILITATION SERVICES:				
5/30	DIET: ADA 1200 Cal.						
	FLUID RESTRICTIONS:						
	TUBE FEEDING:						
	NG TUBE:						
	SUCTION:						
	IRRIGATE:						
	DRAINS/TUBES:		ACTIVITY:		TEACHING:		
			BED REST:				
			BSC:				
			REPOSITION:				
5/30	INTAKE & OUTPUT:		CHAIR:				
	ROUTINE:		UP AD LIB:				
	STRICT:	5/30	AMB. c̄ ASSIST				
	CATHETER: (TYPE)						
	DC ___ ✓ VOIDING	5/30	SIDERAILS:		CENTRAL LINE CARE:		BOWEL/COLOSTOMY CARE:
	IRRIGATION:		☐ FULL ☒ HALF				
			RELEASE SIGNED:				
				6/1	IV SITE: R wrist CHANGE:		
			RESTRAINTS:		IV SITE: CHANGE:		
			☐ WRIST ☐ VEST		IV SITE: CHANGE:		
			☐ 4 PT. LEATHERS				

Figure 23-7A *Kardex*

MODE OF TRANSPORT: AMBULATORY ☒ WHEELCHAIR ☐ CART ☐ BEDSIDE ☐   **MONITOR:** ☐ YES ☐ NO

RESPIRATORY THERAPY	DATE ORD	DATE DONE	MISCELLANEOUS	DATE ORD	DATE DONE	LAB STUDIES	DATE ORD	DAILY STUDIES
O² _____ LPM			ABG'S	5/30		ADMISSION: CBC	5/30	FBS
_____ MASK _____ T-PIECE _____ % O²						CPK/LDH		
_____ VENTILATOR FiO²						CHEM PROF I		
TV _____ RATE						CPK - ISO Q12 HR X 3		
MODE _____ PEEP						6 6 6		
E.T. TUBE SIZE:						6 6		
☐ NASAL ☐ ORAL								
POSITION: cm								
REPOSITIONED: cm								SPECIMEN COLLECTION:
CHANGE/REINSERT								UA ON ADMISSION
SPONTANEOUS PARAMETERS							5/30	
RESP. TX:			EKG STUDIES:	5/30				
			ADMISSION					
X-RAY STUDIES	5/30		Q DAY 3					
CXR ADMISSION								
Q DAY X 3						BLOOD ON HOLD		
						ORD. _____ EXP. _____		

SURGICAL & SPECIAL PROCEDURES	DATE ORD	DATE DONE	CONSULT/REFERRAL	DATE ORD	DATE NOT.	SPEC.
Surgical Fixation ® humerus	6/2		Diabetic teaching	5/30		
PACER: LOCATION		REINSERT:				
CVP: LOCATION		REINSERT:		SOCIAL SERVICE		
A-LINE: LOCATION		REINSERT:		NUTRITIONAL SERVICES		
SWAN: LOCATION		REINSERT:		PATIENT EDUCATION		

ROOM	NAME	AGE	SEX	ADMITTING PHYSICIAN	ADMITTING DIAGNOSIS	RELIGION	ADM. DATE
402	Jayne, Beverly	45	F	Dolster, Wm.	Fx ® humerus		5/30

Figure 23-7B *Kardex*

Charting Practice

Review the guidelines for charting health care records found in Box 2-9 of the textbook. Figure 23-8 is a sample of charting written by a nurse assistant. In the space provided, list 10 of the guidelines for charting that were not followed. Rewrite the information provided in correct form in the space provided.

PATIENT PROGRESS NOTES

DATE	TIME	
5/30	2:30	Mrs. Jayne is an old battleax! She's refusing to eat her meals and complained all day. Her vital signs were okay at 8:15 and 1:30. She has trouble walking unless she's given help because she's so fat. There's some blood on the dressing on her (R) arm —Susie Smith
		TEN GUIDELINES NOT FOLLOWED
	1.	
	2.	
	3.	
	4.	
	5.	
	6.	
	7.	
	8.	
	9.	
	10.	
		CORRECTED VERSION OF CHARTING

*SEE PATIENT PROGRESS NOTES FOR DESCRIPTION.   N/A APPLIES TO NOT APPLICABLE.

Figure 23-8 *Patient progress notes*

The following situations provide informaton for you to record. Chart the necessary information in the space provided in Figure 23-9A and B. Use the charting guidelines found in Chapter 2 of the textbook as reference for the correct method of charting.

PATIENT PROGRESS NOTES

DATE	TIME	

*SEE PATIENT PROGRESS NOTES FOR DESCRIPTION.   N/A APPLIES TO NOT APPLICABLE.

Figure 23-9A *Patient progress notes*

PATIENT PROGRESS NOTES

DATE	TIME	

*SEE PATIENT PROGRESS NOTES FOR DESCRIPTION.   N/A APPLIES TO NOT APPLICABLE.

Figure 23-9B *Patient progress notes*

Situation One

You have been providing care for Mrs. Jameson in room 434, bed 2. Mrs. Jameson is 65 years of age and has been in the hospital for surgery to replace the right hip joint. As you were instructed, you assisted her to walk to the end of the hall four times during your shift. She complained of feeling pain in the hip during the walks and placed a great deal of weight on you during the walks. During the day you assisted Mrs. Jameson to use the bedpan three times. Each time she was able to urinate only a small amount of cloudy foul-smelling urine. She drank a cup of coffee and three glasses of juice during your shift. You also helped Mrs. Jameson take a shower using a shower chair. Mrs. Jameson talked to you several times during the day about her concern about taking care of herself at home when she is discharged, because she lives alone.

Situation Two

You have provided care for Mr. Kennely during your shift. Mr. Kennely is 94 years of age and has pneumonia. He was admitted to the hospital in a confused state of mind. Mr. Kennely does not feed himself so you assisted him to eat breakfast and lunch. He ate about half of both meals. You noticed that Mr. Kennely frequently has a productive cough. The sputum produced is yellowish gray in color. Mr. Kennely left his room and walked to the nurses' lounge during the shift. Once you had discovered that he had left the room, you looked for 5 minutes before finding him there. During the shift you assisted Mr. Kennely with a urinal several times. Mr. Kennely stated repeatedly that he needed to go out and work in his garden. He called you names and swore at you during all of the contacts you had with him.

Applying Your Knowledge

1. In both of the situations, describe any other action you would take in addition to charting your observations.

   _____

   _____

   _____

2. How might you improve the quality of care in each of the patient situations described?

   _____

   _____

   _____

Careers in Nursing

Nursing Skills and Qualities

List three personal qualities and skills that are important in nursing careers.

1. _____

2. _____

3. _____

Identifying Nursing Careers

Use the textbook to complete the missing information about nursing careers in Table 23-1.

TABLE 23-1

Career Title	Years of Education	Description of Job Duties and Opportunities	Credentials Required
		Advanced practice, physical examinations, may prescribe medication, may practice independently	
			LPN, requires licensure
		Supervise the care of patients work in a variety of situations	
	75 hours or more of training		
		Advanced nurse assistant skills in the patient's home	

Applying Your Knowledge

1. Confusion may occur with the background of this professional who might complete a 2-, 3-, or 4-year degree to obtain the same license. This would describe the education of the

   _____.

2. The nurse who may deliver babies is called a _____.

3. An expanded role for the nurse assistant in the community may describe the

   _____.

4. The registered nurse who completes additional training and education may be called a

   _____.

5. The health care worker who works under the supervision of a registered nurse or licensed practical nurse to give daily care is called the _____.

Critical Thinking

Understanding Vital Signs

Figure 23-10 is a sample of a graphic sheet of vital signs for Mrs. Martha Jewel during a 5-day hospital stay.

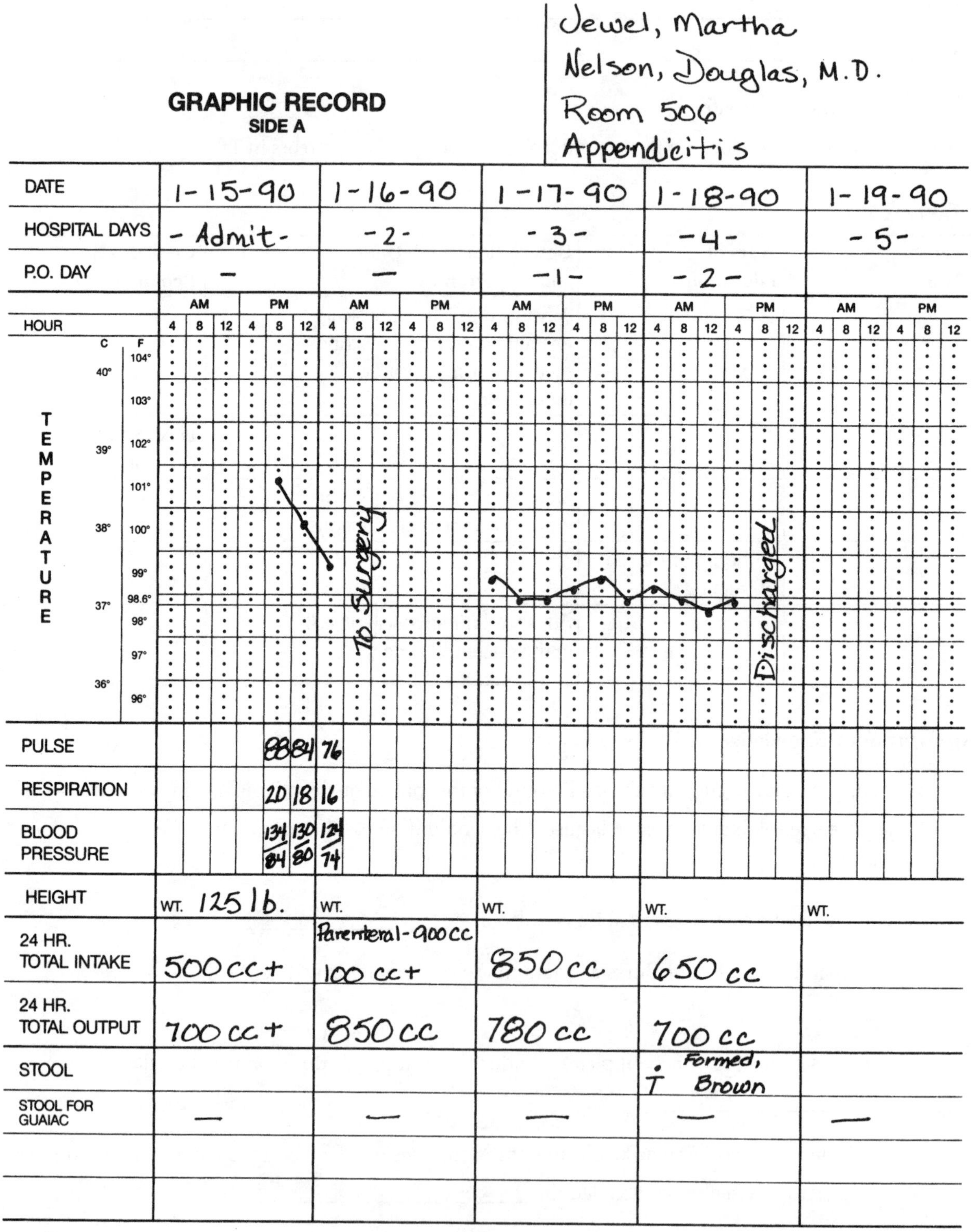

Jewel, Martha
Nelson, Douglas, M.D.
Room 506
Appendicitis

GRAPHIC RECORD
SIDE A

DATE	1-15-90	1-16-90	1-17-90	1-18-90	1-19-90
HOSPITAL DAYS	- Admit -	- 2 -	- 3 -	- 4 -	- 5 -
P.O. DAY	—	—	- 1 -	- 2 -	

PULSE: 88 84 76
RESPIRATION: 20 18 16
BLOOD PRESSURE: 134/84 130/80 124/74
HEIGHT / WT. 125 lb.

24 HR. TOTAL INTAKE	500 cc +	Parenteral - 900 cc 100 cc +	850 cc	650 cc	
24 HR. TOTAL OUTPUT	700 cc +	850 cc	780 cc	700 cc	
STOOL				↑ Formed, Brown	
STOOL FOR GUAIAC	—	—	—	—	—

Figure 23-10

Examining the Evidence

1. Why was Mrs. Jewel admitted to the hospital?

    _____

    _____

    _____

2. When did Mrs. Jewel run a fever during her stay?

    _____

    _____

    _____

3. When was the highest blood pressure reading taken during Mrs. Jewel's stay?

    _____

    _____

    _____

4. On which postoperative day did Mrs. Jewel leave the hospital?

    _____

    _____

    _____

5. When were the vital signs for Mrs. Jewel omitted during her stay?

    _____

    _____

    _____

6. What is the name of Mrs. Jewel's doctor?

    _____

    _____

    _____

24 Medical Careers

Vapid Vocabulary

Before reading the chapter, review the glossary terms from the chapter in the word search puzzle below. Define each of the terms in the space provided.

```
I  P  O  L  T  Y  S  D  C  R  I  I  I  U  Y  R  I  N  H  T
D  I  F  F  E  R  E  N  T  I  A  T  E  R  Y  E  T  I  I  C
V  E  I  Y  V  O  R  O  A  N  N  V  T  O  C  P  R  R  L  O
L  A  N  O  I  T  A  C  O  V  I  R  I  L  I  R  I  I  H  T
E  I  T  G  I  T  A  F  C  S  O  O  O  O  D  E  I  R  D  E
Y  V  O  P  V  R  E  U  N  O  D  E  R  G  E  S  Y  O  T  T
H  C  H  C  I  O  E  E  Y  S  T  Y  T  I  P  C  O  O  Y  R
E  R  H  P  O  O  H  R  A  L  U  C  O  S  O  R  I  V  T  I
E  C  R  I  P  E  T  N  E  R  Y  O  O  T  H  I  V  E  O  I
I  Y  T  A  R  N  T  L  I  P  F  D  D  Y  T  P  L  L  T  T
O  O  P  P  H  O  I  S  Y  O  T  R  P  R  R  T  O  Y  O  I
O  R  M  A  P  I  Y  V  I  T  C  D  L  G  O  I  I  Y  T  N
E  O  C  P  F  T  O  O  O  C  I  L  R  E  I  O  C  F  T  R
C  Y  A  I  N  P  A  O  F  R  I  H  E  I  I  N  I  R  O  Y
O  T  I  V  O  E  E  H  Y  R  A  H  V  I  L  I  D  I  Y  I
I  G  U  I  P  C  T  Y  R  O  C  I  R  D  D  T  R  E  O  C
R  T  Y  O  E  R  L  T  T  N  U  H  T  O  L  T  P  D  R  H
T  E  L  V  P  E  I  C  R  H  I  I  I  R  O  L  R  I  O  T
S  V  O  F  T  P  O  D  I  A  T  R  Y  G  H  I  R  Y  R  R
D  Y  O  R  S  R  D  O  G  D  Y  F  A  T  G  N  D  F  E  A
```

1. Acuity- _____

2. Comprehensive- _____

3. Differentiate- _____

4. Ocular- _____

5. Orthopedic- _____

6. Perception- _____

7. Podiatry- _____

8. Prescription- _____

9. Urologist- _____

10. Vocational- _____

Key Search

Find the Key Terms of the chapter by matching the terms to the definitions in the space provided.

Term Tank		
Acuity	Internship	
Allopathic	Osteopathic	
Anesthesiology	Residency	
Biomechanics	Vision	

DEFINITION	KEY TERM
Period of training in a specific area under the supervision of a qualified health care practitioner	
Treatment of disease and injury with an emphasis on the relationship between body organs and musculoskeletal system	
Clearness or sharpness of perception	
Capacity for sight	
Treatment of disease and injury with active intervention	
Study of the mechanical laws and their application to living organisms, especially locomotion	
Study of medicine to relieve pain during surgery	
Period of initial training under the supervision of a qualified practitioner	

Just the Facts

1. There are two types of medical doctors, the MD (Doctor of _ _ _ _ _ _ _ _) and DO (Doctor of Ⓞ _ _ _ _ _ _ _ _ _ _ Medicine).

2. Additional training under the supervision of a practicing doctor is needed for medical school graduates to specialize and includes an _ _ _ _ _ _ _ _ _ _ _ or

   _ _ _ _ _ _ _ _ _ _.

3. _ _ _ _ _ _ _ _ _ _ _ _ _ _ _ _ _ _ _ are medical doctors who diagnose and treat diseases and injuries to the eyes.

4. The role of the _ _ _ _ _ Ⓞ _ _ _ assistant was developed to relieve some of the tasks performed by the medical doctor to extend the availability of care.

5. Ⓞ _ _ _ _ _ _ _ _ _ _ are eye muscle specialists who work under the direction of an ophthalmologist.

6. _ _ _ _ _ _ _ Ⓞ technologists assist during surgical operations under the supervision of the surgeon and registered nurse.

7. The _ _ _ _ _ _ _ assistant performs both clerical and clinical functions under the supervision of a physician.

8. _ _ _ _ _ _ _ _ _ _ _ _ _ is the ability to differentiate shapes and color to interpret their meaning.

9. The medical or optometric assistant using a _ _ _ _ _ _ _ _ _ _ _ Ⓞ _ that measures the ability to see symbols from a specified distance may test vision.

10. While assisting with the physical examination, the medical assistant may take

    _ _ _ _ _ _ _ _ _ _ _ and _ _ _ _ _ the patient.

Use the circled letters to form the answer to this jumble. Clue: What about a package indicates that it has been sterilized?

_ _ _ _ _

Concept Applications

Reviewing Structures of Anatomy

Use Chapters 9 to 20 to identify each of the structures of the body in Figure 24-1A to E. List the system of the body of which each of the structures is a part and its function in Table 24-1.

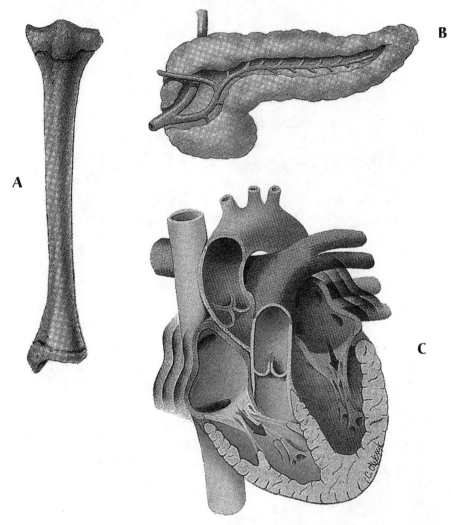

Figure 24-1 Courtesy of Thibodeau: *Anatomy and Physiology*, ed 4, St. Louis, 1999, Mosby.

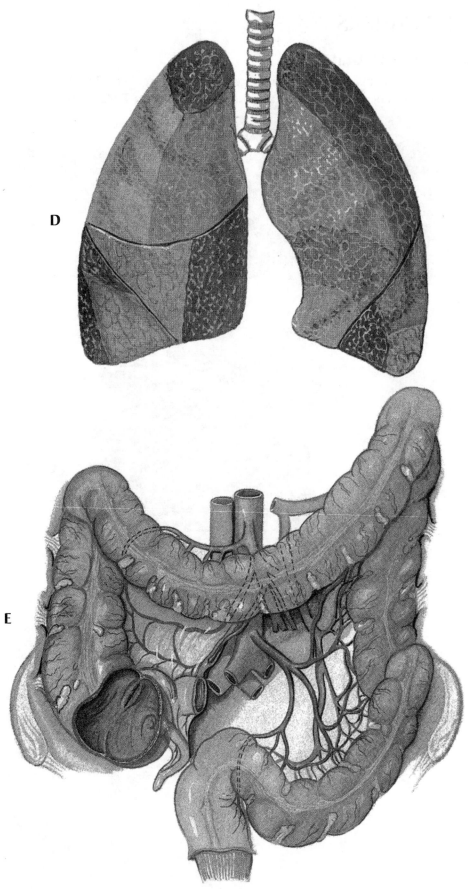

D

E

Figure 24-1 (cont'd)

TABLE 24-1

Body Structure	System	Function
A. _____	_____	_____
B. _____	_____	_____
C. _____	_____	_____
D. _____	_____	_____
E. _____	_____	_____

Medical Careers

List three personal qualities and skills that are important in laboratory careers.

1. _____

2. _____

3. _____

Identifying Medical Careers

Use the textbook to complete the missing information about nursing careers in Table 24-2.

TABLE 24-2

Career Title	Years of Education	Description of Job Duties and Opportunities	Credentials Required
		Use corrective devices, surgery, and medication to treat disorders of the foot	
			OD, licensed by the state
		Anesthesiology, urology, obstetrics, surgery, pediatrics and other specialties; private practice or employment by hospital or clinic	
			DC, licensed by the state
		Work under the supervision of a physician to perform similar duties	

Applying Your Knowledge

1. The health care workers who are eye muscle specialists and who complete 24 months of training following 2 years of college are called _____.

2. A technique that originated with the Chinese and is now performed by health practitioners called _____.

3. The health practitioner who helps the physician and trains for 1 to 2 years is called the _____.

4. Medical doctors who treat disorders of the eyes are called _____.

5. Following licensure or certification by the state, one of the health care practitioners who also must complete at least 100 hours of continuing education every 6 years is called the

_____.

Investigations

Sterilizing Packages

Sterilization is the process used to kill all microorganisms on an object. Read all of the directions before beginning this activity. Laboratory activities should be completed only under the supervision of a qualified professional.

Equipment and Supplies

autoclave
autoclave tape
autoclave paper or lint-free towel
metal instrument for sterilization

Directions

1. Maintain medical asepsis by using good handwashing technique. Wrapping packages for sterilization is a clean procedure requiring that the hands and instruments be as free from microorganisms as possible.

2. Select clean instruments for sterilization. Instruments may be arranged into sets for convenient use in particular procedures.

3. Select a wrapping towel or drape that is large enough to cover all contents completely. Drapes for autoclave sterilization may be made of cotton or specialized disposable material. Draping materials must allow penetration by the pressurized steam or gas.

4. Place instrumentation and sterilizing indicator diagonally in the center of the wrapping material. The outside indicating tape does not ensure that the inner contents have been sterilized.

5. Fold the corners of the draping material into the center of the tray. The near edge is folded first, sides next, and the far side last. The package should be neat and tight with no exposed edges of the wrapping material. Tuck the last edge into the pocket formed by the first three sides.

6. Seal the package with indicator tape. Secure tape so the package will not be pulled open when the tape is removed.

7. Label the tape with the date and time of sterilization, contents, and the initials of the preparer. Items are not considered sterile indefinitely and must be resterilized if not used in a reasonable length of time.

8. Place the package in the appropriate location for articles needing sterilization or load it into the autoclave.

9. Load clean glassware, instruments, or packages into the autoclave with containers and clasps open. Insert indicator tape or pellet. Supplies may be wrapped in muslin, paper, nylon, cellophane, or in a sealing package before sterilization. During autoclaving, closed containers may explode as a result of the expansion of trapped air. Clasps must be opened to allow sterilization of all surface areas. Wrappers must be made of material that allows penetration by the steamed heat.

10. Close and latch the autoclave door.

11. Steam the items for 20 minutes at 20 pounds of pressure at 275° F. The necessary time for steril-ization may differ depending on the size of the load in the autoclave.

12. Allow the pressure of the autoclave to return to zero before opening the door. The pressure read-ing must be at zero before opening the autoclave to avoid rapid release of steam and possible injury.

13. Remove sterile equipment or packages and store them in the appropriate location. Individually sterilized articles must be removed with another sterile instrument to prevent contamination.

Drawing Conclusions

1. Why is it important to place a sterilization indicator inside the package as well as outside?

_____

_____

_____

2. Ethylene oxide gas is used to sterilize materials such as plastics and rubber. Why isn't steam steril-ization used for these materials?

_____

_____

_____

Critical Thinking

Medical Detecting

This activity is adapted from the VQI (Vector Quest I) series developed by the Iowa Medical Founda-tion. It allows you to be an epidemiologist or medical detective. Use the case study to answer the ques-tions.

The Last Case

Janet Parker was very British. She loved tennis at Wimbledon, tea in the afternoon, the Cliffs of Dover, and Monty Python's Flying Circus. In 1978, Ms. Parker died a very un-British death. After becoming severely ill with a high fever and a rash, Ms. Parker died within 5 days. She died from what doctors said could only have been smallpox. Her death was 5 years after Britain had reported its last case of this disease.

Ms. Parker had been a medical photographer employed at the University of Birmingham. One week after Ms. Parker's death, her mother was diagnosed as having the last case of smallpox in Britain. Her mother survived. Neither Janet nor her mother had ever traveled to Africa, where earlier that year the world's last case was prematurely documented.

Regrettably, 1 week after Janet Parker's death, Professor Henry Bedson of the University of Birming-ham committed suicide. Professor Bedson had been the head of the University's Microbiology and Virology Department.

In 1978 the World Health Organization, with help from more than 200,000 health officers and volunteers, won one of mankind's greatest battles. Smallpox was the first disease to be eradicated by human effort. Ironically, Janet Parker, one of its last victims, was from a country that had eradicated the disease years earlier.

Examining the Evidence

1. What questions would you like answered to help determine the source of Janet Parker's illness?

_____

_____

_____

2. Complete the correlation chart in Table 24-3 to determine which variables might be involved in Janet Parker's illness.

_____

_____

_____

TABLE 24-3   CORRELATION CHART

Variable	Significant	Marginal	Low
_____	_____	_____	_____
_____	_____	_____	_____
_____	_____	_____	_____
_____	_____	_____	_____
_____	_____	_____	_____
_____	_____	_____	_____

3. What could have been the vector for Janet Parker's illness?

_____

_____

_____

4. What are four things that can be done by every person to prevent the spread of disease?

_____

_____

_____

5. In your opinion, would it be better to keep or destroy any remaining samples of smallpox that exist?

_____

_____

_____

The Case of the Red Rings

In the summer of 1988 Jeffrey Donner of Waysata, Minnesota was having a typical vacation filled with swimming, cycling, a camping trip with his scout group, a family trip, and baseball. On July 14 of that year, Jeffrey came down with what his family thought was the flu. He had a fever, chills, swollen glands, fatigue, head and body aches, sore throat, and nausea.

Within a 50-mile radius of his home, 78 other people were suffering from the same disease. Ten percent of these people went on to develop cardiac problems, and 15% experienced severe nerve problems.

In talking with Jeffrey it has been discovered that prior to his symptoms he noticed a "ringlike rash" on his lower legs. This bright red mark was approximately 10 cm, or 4 inches wide, and was itchy and painful.

Approximately half of the nearly 80 cases developed arthritic-like conditions within 1 year of the early symptoms. This result was unusual because the victims ranged in age from 3 to 84 years.

Examining the Evidence

1. What questions would you like answered to help determine the source of Jeffrey's illness?

   _____

   _____

   _____

2. Complete the correlation chart in Table 24-4 to determine which variables might be involved in Jeffrey's illness.

   _____

   _____

   _____

TABLE 24-4   CORRELATION CHART

Variable	Significant	Marginal	Low
_____	_____	_____	_____
_____	_____	_____	_____
_____	_____	_____	_____
_____	_____	_____	_____
_____	_____	_____	_____
_____	_____	_____	_____

3. What could have been the vector for Jeffrey's illness?

   _____

   _____

   _____

4. How could the spread of this vector be stopped?

   _____

   _____

   _____

25 *Dental Careers*

Vapid Vocabulary

Before reading the chapter, review the glossary terms from the chapter in the word search puzzle below. Define each of the terms in the space provided.

```
C  I  T  A  M  O  T  P  M  Y  S  A  T  H  R  T  R  E  E  T
N  A  S  S  A  T  R  L  O  L  A  I  E  I  R  E  E  T  A  I
T  S  O  L  T  O  E  O  E  R  E  O  E  E  O  O  E  R  E  T
T  I  A  A  U  T  H  U  T  D  A  U  D  E  T  L  E  O  T  T
R  T  C  H  A  E  A  P  T  A  C  T  I  L  E  S  P  C  M  E
L  A  N  N  C  O  A  A  A  T  H  E  R  M  A  L  O  C  R  D
I  I  O  A  I  I  E  T  G  R  R  T  L  T  L  A  R  U  O  L
E  E  N  Q  T  I  L  E  C  C  G  E  T  E  N  A  O  D  R  Y
N  L  R  Y  E  E  A  T  N  E  I  O  D  S  C  T  O  D  I  E
R  E  E  A  H  S  D  D  U  A  A  O  I  I  A  A  U  E  A  E
P  R  T  L  T  A  C  U  T  E  A  T  T  D  C  U  O  A  U  R
E  U  R  N  S  L  G  Q  P  G  Q  E  I  O  A  U  D  Y  E  E
Y  A  L  I  E  I  R  R  T  D  E  H  S  L  L  R  C  U  T  D
T  E  H  E  T  I  S  I  U  Q  E  R  E  R  P  N  I  N  E  I
E  T  L  R  T  A  D  R  A  S  U  A  R  T  E  A  I  A  I  E
N  N  E  O  A  D  M  R  R  E  D  P  T  C  R  R  O  E  Q  D
E  D  I  R  O  U  L  F  T  O  E  R  E  O  I  I  Q  C  E  T
D  T  T  U  T  E  T  C  D  O  I  T  H  A  E  I  O  I  T  E
E  D  O  T  C  S  T  D  F  L  R  E  C  O  T  P  U  N  T  O
R  A  T  C  T  T  E  T  S  E  E  S  T  N  E  O  O  A  E  C
```

1. Acute- _____

2. Asymptomatic- _____

3. Esthetic- _____

4. Fluoride- _____

   5. Inlay- _____

   6. Neonate- _____

   7. Prerequisite- _____

   8. Radiograph- _____

   9. Tactile- _____

 10. Thermal- _____

Key Search

Find the Key Terms of the chapter by matching the terms to the definitions in the space provided.

Term Tank			
Abscess	Caries	Halitosis	Periodontal
Alloy	Deciduous	Hygiene	Permanent
Alveoli	Dentition	Mandible	Plaque
Calculus	Gingiva	Maxilla	Restoration

DEFINITION	KEY TERM
Gum of the mouth; mucous membrane with supporting fibrous tissue	
Bone of the lower jaw	
Replacement of part of a tooth, usually with silver alloy, gold, or esthetic composite material	
Bony cavities in maxilla and mandible in which the roots of the teeth are attached	
Solid mixture of two or more metals	
Mass adhering to the enamel surface of a tooth, composed of mixed bacterial colonies and organic material	
Situated or occurring around a tooth	
Calcium phosphate and carbonate with organic matter, deposited on the surfaces of teeth; tartar	
Localized collection of pus in a cavity formed by destruction of tissue	
Decalcification on the surface of the tooth followed by disintegration of the inner part of the tooth; cavity	

Continued

DEFINITION	KEY TERM
The teeth that erupt first and are replaced by permanent dentition; primary teeth	
Used to designate natural teeth in the mouth	
Proper care of the mouth and teeth for maintenance of health and the prevention of disease	
Irregularly shaped bone that forms the upper jaw	
Offensive or bad breath	
The teeth that erupt and take the palce of deciduous dentition; secondary teeth	

Just the Facts

1. The dental team includes the _ _ _ _ _ ○ _, dental _ _ _ _ _ _ _ _ _ _, dental _ _ _ _ _ ○ _ _ _, and dental _ _ _ _ _ _ _ _ _ _ _ technician.

2. Dentists perform a variety of services including _ _ _ _ _ _ education, detection of ○ _ _ _ _ _ _ _, _ _ _ _ _ _ _ _ _ improvement of appearance, and correction of ○ _ _ _ problems.

3. Some of the _ _ _ _ _ specialties that dentists may practice include endodontics, orthodontics, and periodontics.

4. Some areas in which the dental _ _ _ ○ _ _ _ _ _ may specialize include clinical work, education, administration, research, consumer advocacy, or veterinary dental practice.

5. The dental _ _ _ _ _ _ _ _ _'_ responsibilities may include answering the telephone, making appointments, and working with billing accounts.

6. Dental _ _ _ ○ _ _ _ _ _ _ _ _ ○ _ _ _ _ _ _ _ _ _ are the only members of the dental health care team who do not work directly with patients.

7. ○ _ _ _ _ _ _ _ _ _ disease is caused by infection in the supporting structures of teeth such as the gingiva and bones.

8. Functions of the teeth include the mechanical portion of _ _ _ _ _ _ _ _ _, _ _ _ _ _ of the face, and aid in the production of _ _ ○ _ _ _.

9. The tooth is divided into two sections called the _ _ _ _ ◯ and _ _ _ _ _.

10. Descriptive anatomy of the tooth is called _ ◯ _ _ _ _ _ _ _ _ _.

Use the circled letters to form the answer to this jumble. Clue: What is the practice of dentistry that provides care for children?

_ _ _ _ _ _ _ _ _ _ _ _ _ _

Concept Applications

Identifying Structures of the Oral Cavity

Use Figure 25-6 in the textbook to label the diagram of the oral cavity in Figure 25-1.

tongue   uvula   upper lip
lower lip   hard palate   soft palate

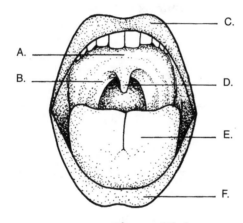

Figure 25-1

A. _____   D. _____
B. _____   E. _____
C. _____   F. _____

Identifying Structures of the Tooth

Use Figure 25-8 in the textbook to label the diagram of the tooth in Figure 25-2.

crown   pulp   dentin
root   enamel

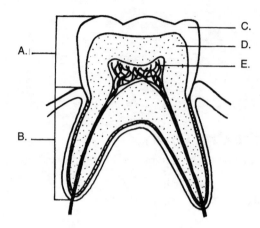

Figure 25-2

A. _____   D. _____

B. _____   E. _____

C. _____

Identifying Teeth in the Mouth

Use Figure 25-7 in the textbook to label the diagram of the teeth in the mouth in Figure 25-3.

mandibular teeth	maxillary teeth	cuspid
central incisor	lateral incisor	bicuspid
first molar	second molar	third molar

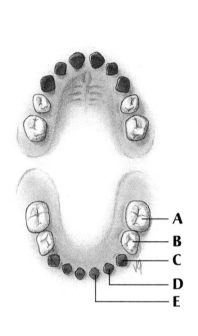

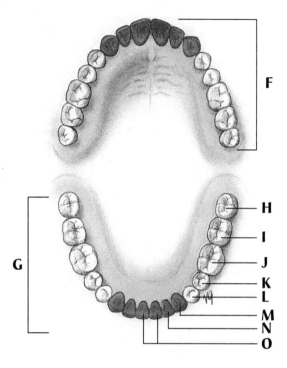

Figure 25-3

A. _____   I. _____

B. _____   J. _____

C. _____   K. _____

D. _____   L. _____

E. _____   M. _____

F. _____   N. _____

G. _____   O. _____

H. _____

Identifying the Surfaces of the Teeth

Use Figure 25-9 in the textbook to label the diagram of the tooth surfaces in Figure 25-4.

buccal   mesial   lingual
distal   occlusal

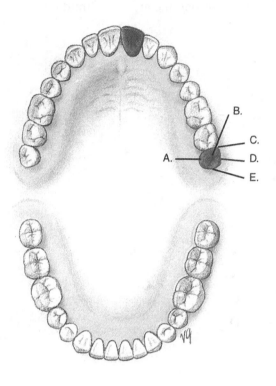

Figure 25-4

A. _____   D. _____

B. _____   E. _____

C. _____

Charting Dental Structures

Mrs. Smith is a 62-year-old. She has the following dental history. Use Figure 25-10 in the textbook to chart the information regarding Mrs. Smith's dentition in Figure 25-5.

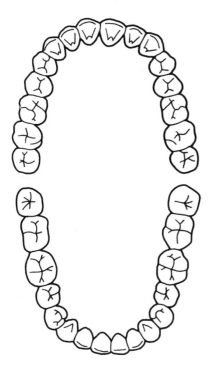 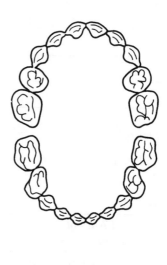

Figure 25-5

TABLE 25-1

Tooth Number	Dental Structure
1	Tooth missing
2	Amalgam restoration
3	Amalgam restoration
14	Esthetic restoration
15	Gold crown
16	Tooth missing
17	Amalgam restoration
18	Caries or decay
31	Root canal
32	Gold crown

Drawing Conclusions

1. Why is it normal for the third molars to be missing?

_____

_____

_____

2. Why would Mrs. Smith need a dental visit?

_____

_____

_____

Dental Careers

Dental Skills and Qualities

List three personal qualities and skills that are important in dental careers.

1. _____

2. _____

3. _____

Identifying Dental Careers

Use the textbook to complete the missing information about dental careers in Table 25-2.

TABLE 25-2

Career Title	Years of Education	Description of Job Duties and Opportunities	Credentials Required
	No educational standards set, 1 to 2 years of training		
			DDS or DMD, licensure required
		Scope of practice varies greatly; clean teeth, record patient history, take radiographs, teach dental hygiene, administer anesthesia	

Applying Your Knowledge

1. The health care worker who applies braces to correct misalignment of teeth is called a

   _____.

2. The health care worker who gives instruction on how to floss teeth is the

   _____.

3. Dental radiographs may be taken by two different workers including the

   _____ and the _____.

4. The health care worker who cleans the teeth below the gum is the _____.

5. After an accident, surgery to correct injuries would probably be completed by the

   _____.

EKG

9ᵗʰ-10ᵗʰ. Read Chat. 29
W Pt. Case As gist Complete questions
in back of the Chat.

Other Info neeleD for EKG → CV system
Chpt. H, pg. 383 in theo Teem text

CARDIO

Investigations

Practicing Oral Hygiene

Read all of the directions before beginning this activity. Laboratory activities should be completed only under the supervision of a qualified professional.

Equipment and Supplies

dental floss
disclosing tablet
mirror
toothbrush
toothpaste

Directions

1. Practice medical asepsis by using good handwashing technique.

2. Brush your teeth for 3 minutes using a toothbrush and toothpaste of preference.

3. Floss your teeth as instructed in the textbook.

4. Chew a disclosing tablet provided by your instructor.

5. Use a mirror to identify the areas missed during brushing and flossing.

6. Brush your teeth to remove all color remaining from the tablet.

Drawing Conclusions

1. Which areas of your teeth, if any, did you omit in the brushing?

   _____

   _____

   _____

2. Why would it be more likely for a cavity to form on a tooth that is habitually missed during brushing?

   _____

   _____

   _____

Practicing Dental Identification

Read all of the directions before beginning this activity. Laboratory activities should be completed only under the supervision of a qualified professional.

Equipment and Supplies

dental floss
toothbrush
toothpaste

Directions

1. Practice medical asepsis by using good handwashing technique.

2. Brush and floss your teeth using the instructions in the textbook.

3. With a partner, use the instruction in the textbook to chart each student's dental history in Figure 25-6.

4. Hold your mouth open widely for another student to see and chart the dental structures and restorations visible. You may use your fingers to hold your mouth open widely. NOTE: Each student only places his or her fingers in his/or own mouth.

Drawing Conclusions

1. Why does each student place his or her own fingers into his or her own mouth?

   _____

   _____

   _____

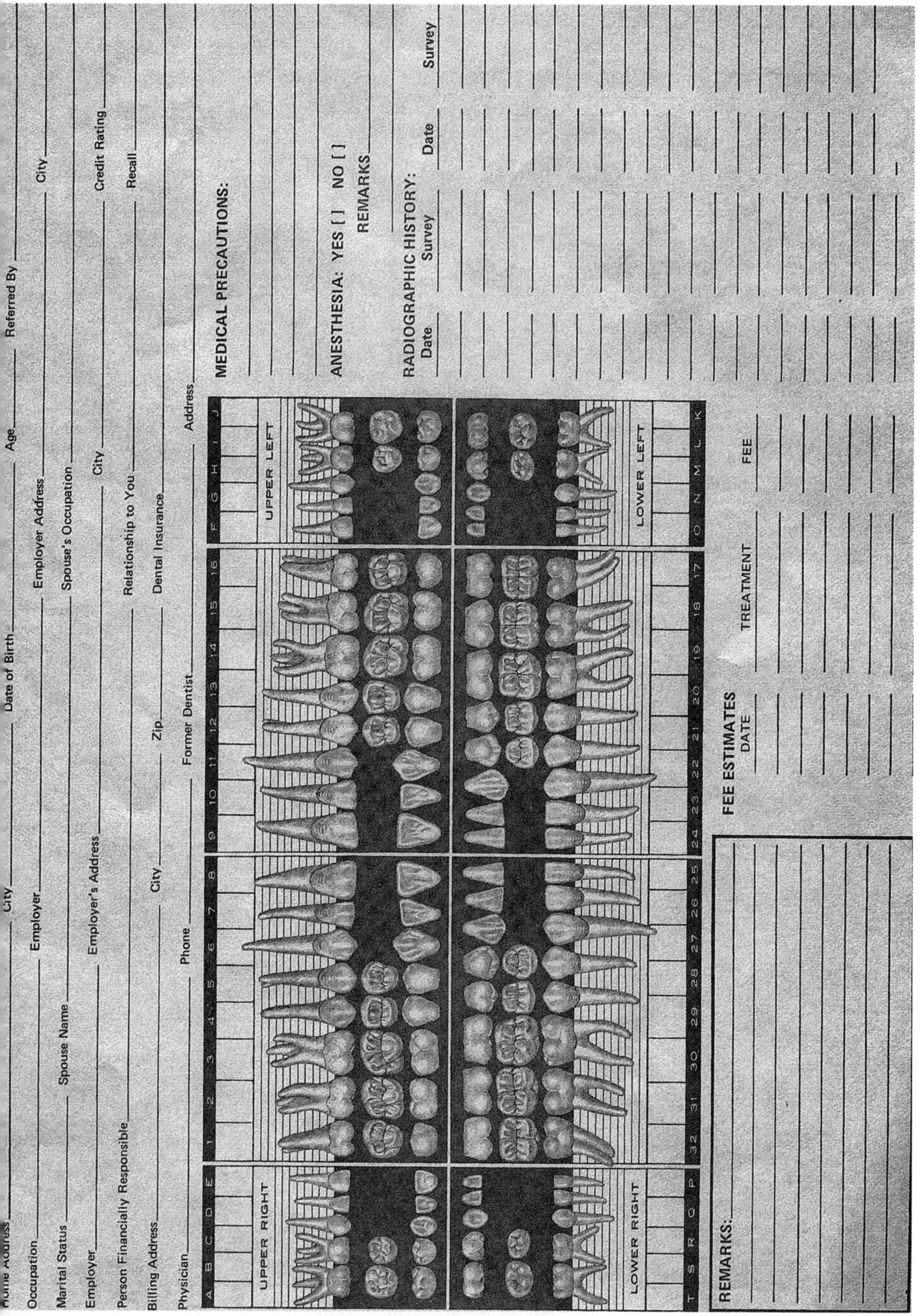

Figure 25-6A *Dental history form (Courtesy of Professional Publishers)*

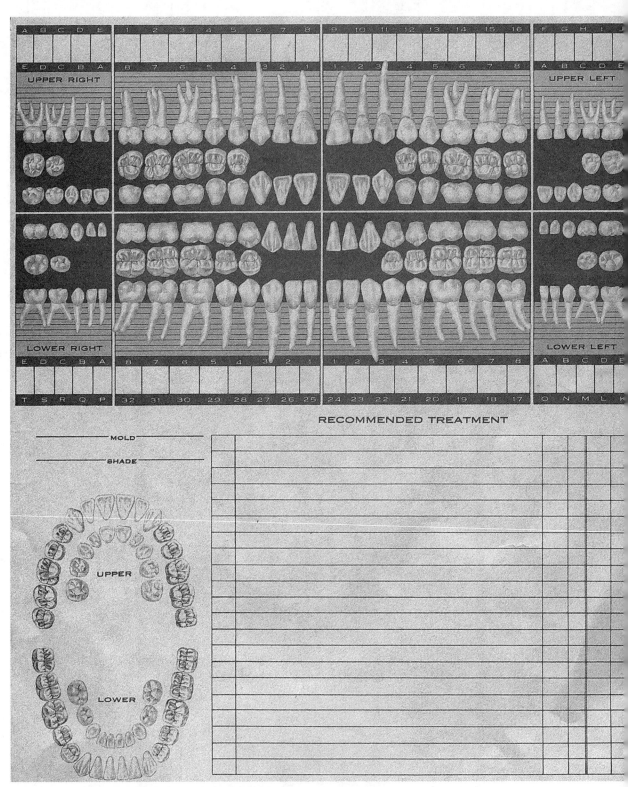

Figure 25-6B *Dental history form (Courtesy of Professional Publishers)*

Critical Thinking

Dental Phobia

More than an estimated 40 million Americans suffer from some degree of "dental phobia," or an irrational fear of dental examination. Symptoms of this problem include anxiety and physiologic changes related to stress. Some techniques have been developed to reduce the phobia related to dental appointments, including resisting the negative thoughts about the visit before seeing the dentist. It has also been demonstrated that it may be helpful for the patient to focus on taking regular breaths during the visit and to inform the dentist when fear is present. Focusing on positive thoughts such as "I am getting good care and improving my health" also may be helpful.

Examining the Evidence

1. Why do you think some people experience dental phobia?

   _____

   _____

   _____

2. What other suggestions could you make to reduce the anxiety of the dental visit?

   _____

   _____

   _____

3. What could a health care worker do in the office to reduce the dental phobia of the patient?

   _____

   _____

   _____

4. What other statements could be used to generate positive thoughts and promote concentration during the appointment?

   _____

   _____

   _____

5. Why is it important to communicate the fear of a dental visit to the dentist?

   _____

   _____

   _____

Gum is Good?

Some types of chewing gum actually help to prevent tooth decay. Xylitol, a sweetener made from cornstalks, helps to seal caries. A 3-year study to test the role of xylitol in tooth decay involving 1200 children between the ages of 9 and 11 years was conducted by Kauko K. Makinen, a biochemist at the University of Michigan, who reached this conclusion. The experiment involved having the children chew gum three to five times a day for several minutes. Some gums used contained xylitol, whereas others contained sucrose (sugar) or sorbitol (another artificial sweetener).

The study showed a slightly higher increase in tooth decay in children who chewed gum with sucrose than in those who did not chew gum at all. Both of these graphs showed a higher increase in the number of caries than in the children chewing gum with sorbitol. However, a comparable *decrease* was found in the number of caries in children chewing gum with xylitol.

Makinen also reported that bacteria that cause caries do not break down xylitol into acids. Because the xylitol is not broken down into acids, the bacteria then do not cause decay.

Examining the Evidence

1. What controls did Makinen use in the study concerning gum sweeteners?

   _____

   _____

   _____

2. How could this study be duplicated?

   _____

   _____

   _____

3. Visualize and describe an advertisement for print or audio to sell a gum containing xylitol.

   _____

   _____

   _____

4. In more than one mystery story, the culprit is caught by matching the indentations of his or her teeth that were found at the scene of the crime, in foods such as cheese or even gum. Is this a realistic scenario?

   _____

   _____

   _____

Complementary and Alternative Careers

26

Vapid Vocabulary

Before reading the chapter, review the glossary terms from the chapter in the word search puzzle below. Define each of the terms in the space provided.

```
Y  E  V  I  T  A  N  R  E  T  L  A  I  E  A  M  T  D  X  O
T  R  E  V  I  T  A  R  G  E  T  N  I  N  R  C  T  C  E  E
I  E  A  P  N  I  M  I  A  I  A  O  E  E  H  A  T  V  C  A
I  E  H  T  E  O  A  L  N  R  O  N  O  R  L  C  I  C  E  C
M  G  O  A  N  P  S  Y  C  H  O  S  O  M  A  T  I  C  A  N
L  P  I  H  E  E  R  X  L  I  I  N  A  R  A  L  D  M  I  B
A  C  L  E  L  L  M  T  Y  N  I  I  T  L  R  M  R  N  L  R
T  M  V  R  V  N  H  E  A  C  T  X  U  I  E  N  O  I  N  L
X  N  U  B  M  R  V  N  L  N  E  P  C  M  A  T  O  R  V  A
C  M  I  A  X  H  L  D  M  P  I  M  L  L  A  M  I  L  T  E
A  N  O  L  E  E  O  N  M  N  M  M  B  L  A  N  N  I  R  X
S  E  I  D  E  M  E  R  A  N  M  O  E  N  C  L  E  C  H  C
A  I  L  R  I  N  M  M  I  I  R  M  C  N  R  A  E  N  M  O
A  B  L  H  C  R  L  H  P  N  O  A  L  M  A  C  Y  E  I  C
L  I  B  E  H  T  X  I  I  L  L  I  H  E  N  V  M  V  O  E
M  H  V  I  L  N  Y  N  T  D  C  V  E  P  R  H  I  H  I  O
T  M  N  M  V  L  Y  M  M  I  E  I  B  M  N  M  L  M  M  D
C  I  I  A  P  L  M  E  H  T  A  E  L  I  I  R  L  A  X  O
N  I  C  M  A  E  L  M  R  E  N  P  P  L  E  I  N  X  L  I
H  D  N  T  V  A  R  N  R  E  R  E  H  P  A  R  I  D  M  I
```

1. Alternative- _____

2. Chronic- _____

3. Complementary- _____

4. Extract- _____

5. Herbal- _____

6. Integrative- _____

7. Manipulative- _____

8. Melatonin- _____

9. Psychosomatic- _____

10. Remedies- _____

Key Search

Find the Key Terms of the chapter by matching the terms to the definitions in the space provided.

Term Tank		
Allopathic	Homeopathic	
Biofeedback	Hydrotherapy	
Chiropractic	Subluxation	
Holistic		

DEFINITION	KEY TERM
System of medical practice that uses remedies designed to product similar effects to those caused by the disease being treated	
External use of water to treat disease	
Conscious control of biological functions normally controlled involuntarily	
Incomplete dislocation of a joint	
Practice of medicine that considers the person as a whole unit, not as individual parts	
System of therapy based on the theory that health is determined by the condition of the nervous system	
System of medical practice that uses remedies designed to product effects that are different than those caused by the disease being treated	

Just the Facts

1. Complementary medicine is a therapy based on _ _ _ _ _ _ _ _ and
   _ _ Ⓞ _ _ _ _ treatment.

2. Based on information gathered in a 1997 survey, the *Journal of the American Medical Association* reported that more than 42% of Americans use therapies outside of
   _ _ _ _ _ _ _ Ⓞ _ _ _ medicine.

3. The National Institutes of Health groups CAM practices into _ _ Ⓞ _
   _ _ _ _ _ _ _ _.

4. _ _ _ _ _ _ _ _ _ _ _ Ⓞ _ _ _ treat health problems associated with the muscular, skeletal, and nervous system.

5. Ⓞ _ _ _ _ _ _ _ _ _ _ _ _ doctors are primary care physicians that focus on treatment of the whole person with emphasis on wellness and disease prevention.

6. _ _ _ _ _ _ Ⓞ _ _ _ _ _ _ _ _ _ Ⓞ _ _ _ use skillful touch to loosen muscles and relieve pain.

7. _ _ _ _ _ _ _ _ _ _ _ _ _ _ _ insert needles into peripheral or surface nerves to control pain, provide anesthesia, relieve symptoms, and modify psychosomatic disorders.

8. _ Ⓞ _ _ _ _ _ _ _ _ _ is a technique used to change normally involuntary reactions of the body using conscious control.

9. _ _ _ _ _ _ Ⓞ _ _ _ _ medicine is a Western system based on the concept that "like cures like."

10. Many of the biologically based therapies that are considered to be CAM overlap with conventional medicine and involve special _ _ Ⓞ _ _ _ _ _
    _ _ _ _ _ _ _ Ⓞ _ _ _ or programs.

Use the circled letters to form the answer to this jumble. Clue: What are the nonallopathic practices that have been proven to be effective by research called?

_ _ _ _ _ _ _ _ _ _ _ _

Concept Applications

Describing the Domains of CAM

In the space below, describe each of the five domains of complementary and alternative medicine.

1. Alternative medical systems:

_____

_____

_____

2. Manipulative and body-based methods:

_____

_____

_____

3. Mind-body interventions:

_____

_____

_____

4. Biological-based theory:

_____

_____

_____

5. Energy therapy:

_____

_____

_____

Complementary and Alternative Careers

Complementary and Alternative Skills and Qualities

List three personal qualities and skills that are important in complementary and alternative careers.

1. _____

2. _____

3. _____

Identifying Complementary and Alternative Careers

Use the textbook to complete the missing information about complementary and alternative careers in Table 26-1.

TABLE 26-1

Career Title	Years of Education	Description of Job Duties and Opportunities	Credentials Required
	Minimum of 2 years of college and completion of a 4- to 5-year program		
		Application of needles into peripheral nerves to control pain, provide anesthesia, and relieve symptoms	
Naturopathic doctor			
			Licensure required in 13 states
			Certification available for applicants licensed or working under the supervision of a licensed health care practitioner

Applying Your Knowledge

1. The practitioner that adjusts the spine to correct disorders is the _____.

2. A practitioner who helps the patient overcome bad habits and treats emotional problems is the

   _____.

3. The CAM practitioner that holds a medical degree but does not prescribe medications is the

   _____   _____.

4. The CAM practitioner that uses a technique believed to release endorphins into the bloodstream is

   the _____.

5. Manipulation of the skin, muscles, tendons, and ligaments is a therapeutic technique of the

   _____   _____.

Investigations

Using Biofeedback to Measure and Control Body Reactions

Read all of the instructions before beginning this activity. Laboratory activities should be completed only under the supervision of a qualified professional

Equipment and Supplies

Liquid crystal thermal indicator (Biodot)

Directions

1. Wash and dry both hands thoroughly

2. Apply a liquid crystal thermal indicator to the flap between the thumb and index finger on the hand that is not dominant.

3. Note the color of the Biodot in Table 26-2

4. Monitor the color of the Biodot throughout the rest of the day, noting the time and activity of any color change. Data collection is completed when the Biodot becomes dislodged.

5. Record the information in Table 26-2 for any color change that occurs.

TABLE 26–2

Time of Reading	Color of Biodot	Activity
Initial =		

Questions

1. What type of activity was the most stressful using the biodot as the indicator of your stress level?

   _____

   _____

   _____

2. Did you feel most stressed during the activity indicated to be stressful according to the biodot?

   _____

   _____

   _____

3. What are some other factors that might influence the reading of the biodot?

_____

_____

_____

4. What are some other measurements that could indicate increased stress that would be more reliable than the Biodot?

_____

_____

_____

5. What type of relaxation technique could you use during stressful activities?

_____

_____

_____

Critical Thinking

Understanding Clinical Trials

Using the Internet link below, read about clinical trials in CAM being conducted by the National Institutes of Health.

http://nccam.nih.gov/clinicaltrials/factsheet/index.htm

Answer the following questions:

1. What is a clinical trial?

_____

_____

_____

2. What are the common elements of a clinical trial?

_____

_____

_____

3. What is a placebo?

_____

_____

_____

4. What are the benefits and risks of participating in a clinical trial?

_____

_____

_____

Using the Internet link below, investigate a CAM clinical trial being conducted by the National Institutes of Health. Complete the information in Table 26-3.

http://nccam.nih.gov/clinicaltrials/

TABLE 26-3

Description of study	
Eligibility criteria for participants	
Length of study	
Location of organization or parties completing the study	
Domain of Cam	

Write a paragraph that describes the clinical trial. Include the purpose (intended outcome), supporting data, and your evaluation of the method being studied.

_____

_____

_____

_____

_____

_____

27 Veterinary Careers

Vapid Vocabulary

Before reading the chapter, review the glossary terms from the chapter in the word search puzzle below. Define each of the terms in the space provided.

```
I  C  I  T  S  E  M  O  D  A  U  S  R  I  A  N  C  I  E  T
N  M  U  E  Y  N  S  N  Y  I  R  E  T  I  A  N  R  I  M  T
C  I  E  I  A  V  O  T  I  A  I  S  R  I  T  N  U  R  T  I
I  S  B  O  T  R  I  T  E  M  S  E  M  N  I  A  Y  S  M  N
N  N  A  E  N  N  I  I  E  T  A  E  T  E  M  R  Y  U  S  N
E  O  N  S  I  S  N  E  T  I  A  M  N  N  U  A  I  O  B  B
R  A  T  L  N  E  T  E  A  E  E  S  T  V  M  V  N  I  M  I
A  T  A  E  E  N  E  T  M  N  I  A  R  T  S  E  R  C  V  S
T  S  E  S  S  I  Y  I  I  E  E  N  M  I  N  R  E  I  N  I
E  E  B  M  C  B  A  N  N  R  N  C  M  S  C  S  M  V  U  V
R  R  E  I  E  A  N  N  A  M  N  A  V  R  E  U  S  M  N  R
I  T  R  R  T  E  L  I  N  T  N  S  S  E  T  R  O  D  E  A
S  A  I  V  S  N  T  E  I  T  O  I  M  R  Y  R  R  S  A  I
Y  T  I  R  E  T  X  E  D  I  O  B  E  N  I  R  A  M  I  I
C  R  M  A  C  B  R  M  N  S  I  M  I  A  O  T  I  R  E  C
I  R  A  M  E  M  R  T  R  C  R  V  O  I  I  N  O  T  S  I
R  I  N  S  N  N  I  I  V  A  M  S  T  R  S  R  E  I  T  N
R  U  R  A  L  N  E  O  Y  E  S  I  V  V  S  I  V  A  I  A
I  M  N  V  L  E  B  A  E  E  I  S  R  E  I  S  N  E  C  R
O  T  S  I  E  I  S  U  E  R  N  N  E  I  M  R  A  T  E  M
```

1. Botany- _____

2. Dexterity- _____

3. Domestic- _____

4. Inanimate- _____

5. Incinerate- _____

6. Marine- _____

7. Restrain- _____

8. Rural- _____

9. Salinity- _____

10. Vicious- _____

Key Search

Find the Key Terms of the chapter by matching the terms to the definitions in the space provided.

Term Tank		
Bovine	Feline	Theriogenology
Canine	Immunize	Vaccination
Carcass	Parasite	Veterinary
Equine	Quarantine	

DEFINITION	KEY TERM
Plant or animal that lives on or within another living organism at the expense of the host organism	
Pertaining to cattle	
Introduction of a microorganism that has been made harmless into a human or animal for the purpose of developing immunity	
Secure against a particular disease	
Pertaining to dogs	
Pertaining to cats	
Branch of veterinary medicine dealing with reproduction	
Dead body of an animal	
Period of detention or isolation as a result of a disease suspected to be communicable	
Pertaining to horses	
Pertaining to animals and their diseases	

Just the Facts

1. Veterinary care personnel work in a variety of settings including _ O _ _ _ _ _ practice, O _ _ _ _ _ _ health, _ _ O _ _ _ _ _ _, zoos, and racetracks.

2. Three of the 16 recognized board specialties for veterinarians are
   _ _ _ _ _ _ _ _ _ _ _ O _ _ _ _, ophthalmology, and _ _ _ _
   medicine.

3. Three out of four veterinarians work in private practice with either _ _ _ _ _ or
   _ _ _ _ _ animals.

4. _ _ _ _ _ _ _ _ or marine biologists study plant and animal life in saltwater environments.

5. Common pets include dogs, cats, turtles, O _ _ _ _, fish, small
   _ _ O _ _ _ _, horses, and O _ _ _ _ _ _.

6. _ _ O _ _ _ _ _ _ _ is the process of surgical sterilization to prevent unwanted
   births.

7. Induction of death in a sick, severely injured, or unwanted animal is called
   _ _ _ _ _ _ _ _ O _ _.

8. _ O _ _ _ _ _ _ _ _ _ for physically and mentally ill people is rapidly becoming an accepted treatment method in many health care settings.

9. More than 150 diseases called _ _ _ _ _ _ _ O _ can be transmitted from animals to
   humans.

10. Some indications that an animal is sick include abnormal behavior, especially sudden
    _ _ _ _ O _ _ _ _ _ _ or O _ _ _ _ _ _ _ _ _ _ _ _,
    and abnormal discharge from any body opening.

Use the circled letters to form the answer to this jumble. Clue: What is one vital sign that may be low-
ered as a benefit of pet therapy?

_ _ _ _ _ _   _ _ _ _ _ _ _ _

Concept Applications

Identifying Animal Restraints

Use Figure 27-6 in the textbook to label the diagram of the animal restraints in Figure 27-1.

    chute   snare   muzzle
    twitch   bag

A.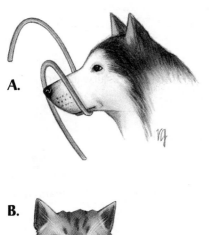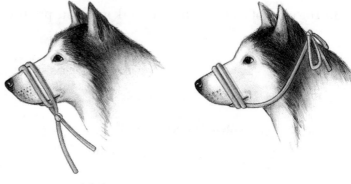

B. 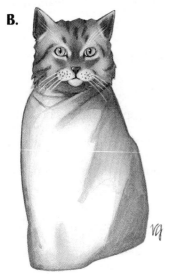   **C.**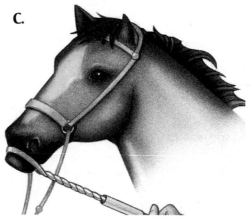

Figure 27-1

D.

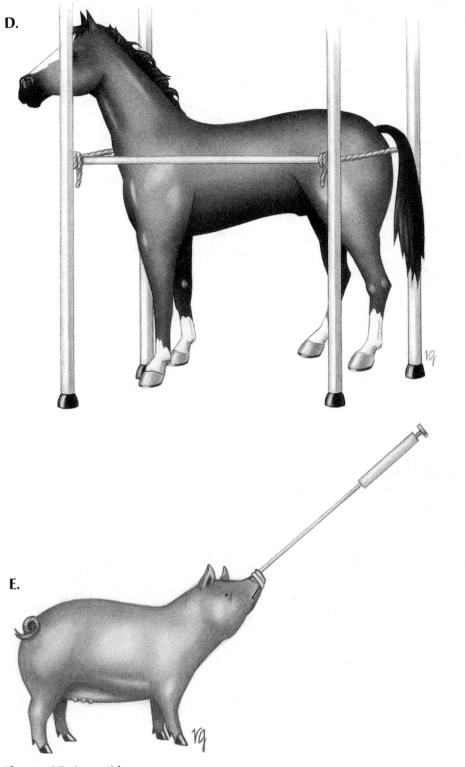

E.

Figure 27-1 cont'd

A. _____   D. _____

B. _____   E. _____

C. _____

Identifying Sites for Blood Collection

Use Figure 27-7 in the textbook to label the diagram of the blood collection sites in Figure 27-2.

saphenous vein   cephalic vein
femoral vein   jugular vein

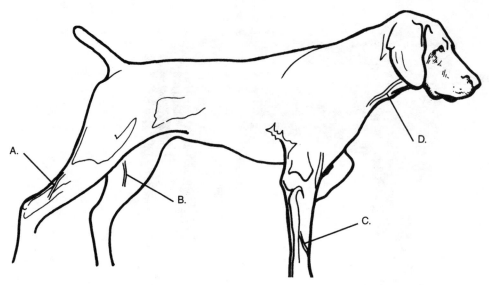

Figure 27-2

Identifying Disorders of Animals

Use the textbook to complete the missing information about animal disorders in Table 27-1. Note the etiology (causing factor), signs and symptoms, and treatment and method of prevention (if any).

Applying Your Knowledge

1. The animal disorder that can be found in humans as well as animals and is usually fatal is called

   _____.

2. The disorder that appears in calves and is caused by bacteria in a soiled environment is called

   _____.

3. The viral infection affecting cats that involves inflammation of the nose and trachea is called

   _____.

4. The condition that affects dogs and is transmitted by mosquitoes is called

   _____.

5. The condition that may occur in horses that lick flies from their hair is called

   _____.

TABLE 27-1

Disorder	Etiology	Signs and Symptoms	Treatment and Prevention
	Virus found in fecal waste	Affects dogs	
	Feeding mismanagement, worms	Affects horses	
		Affects cats	Vaccination; supportive measures to counteract signs; quarantine; death results if untreated
		Affects cats; painful, frequent urination, blood in urine, depression, death	
		Affects dogs	Self-limiting, antiotics if bronchopneumonia develops
	Virus transmitted in saliva		
	Microorganisms transferred by dairy equipment		

Animal Health Careers

Animal Health Skills and Qualities

List three personal qualities and skills that are important in animal health careers.

1. _____

2. _____

3. _____

Identifying Animal Health Careers

Use the textbook to complete the missing information about animal health careers in Table 27-2.

TABLE 27-2

Career Title	Years of Education	Description of Job Duties and Opportunities	Credentials Required
		Research on ocean life; work in ecology; usually employed by universities, private industry or the government	
			DVM or VMD, licensed by the state
		Research, food inspection, laboratory or private clinic; prepare and test vaccines, collect specimens, administer medication	
	On-the-job training or home study		
		Use genetic traits to meet breeding needs of owners	

Applying Your Knowledge

1. The professional who might specialize in practice with small or large animals is the

   _____.

2. Extended duties such as teeth cleaning, removal of sutures, and administration of intravenous fluids may be learned by the _____.

3. To obtain a cow that produces more milk, the dairy farmer may consult an

   _____.

4. Environmental conditions such as soil and water salinity and temperature may be studied by the

   _____.

Investigations

Performing an Animal Health Assessment

Read all of the instructions before beginning this activity. Laboratory activities should be completed only under the supervision of a qualified professional

Equipment and Supplies

domestic animal such as a cat or dog
stethoscope

Directions

1. Maintain medical asepsis by practicing frequent handwashing when handling animals.

2. Restrain the animal as needed to prevent injury to yourself or the animal.

3. Observe the animal to complete the assessment form in Figure 27-3. Use caution to avoid injury to yourself or the animal.

4. Complete the temperature assessment and anal sac examination only under the supervision of a qualified animal care professional.

5. Release and reward the animal with affection.

6. Clean and replace equipment to the designated location.

Pet's name: _____

Owner's name: _____

Species: _____ Breed: _____

Sex: _____ Age: _____ Weight _____ Temp: _____

Exam date: _____ By: _____

Examination Checklist

Coat and Skin

___ Appear normal   ___ Matted
___ Dull   ___ Tumors

Coat and Skin (cont.)

___ Scaly   ___ Itchy
___ Dry   ___ Parasites
___ Oily   ___ Other _____
___ Shedding   _____

Recommendation: _____

Eyes

___ Appear normal   ___ Infection
___ Discharge   ___ Cataract ___ L ___ R
___ Inflamed   ___ Other _____
___ Eyelid deformity   _____

Recommendation: _____

Figure 27-3

Examination Checklist continued

Ears

___ Appear normal   ___ Tumor ___ L ___ R
___ Inflamed   ___ Excessive hair
___ Itchy   ___ Other _____
___ Mites   _____

Recommendation: _____

Nose and Throat

___ Appear normal   ___ Inflamed tonsils
___ Nasal discharge   ___ Enlarged glands
___ Inflamed throat   ___ Other _____

Recommendation: _____

Mouth, Teeth, and Gums

___ Appear normal   ___ Inflamed lips
___ Broken teeth   ___ Loose teeth
___ Tartar buildup   ___ Pyorrhea
___ Tumors   ___ Other _____
___ Ulcers   _____

Recommendation: _____

Legs and Paws

___ Appear normal   ___ Joint disorder
___ Lameness   ___ Nail disorder
___ Damaged ligaments   ___ Other _____
___ Shedding   _____

Recommendation: _____

Heart

___ Appear normal   ___ Fast
___ Murmur   ___ Other _____
___ Slow   _____

Recommendation: _____

Abdomen

___ Appears normal   ___ Abnormal mass
___ Enlarged organs   ___ Tense or painful
___ Fluid   ___ Other _____
                            _____

Recommendation: _____

Lungs

___ Appear normal   ___ Difficulty breathing
___ Abnormal sound   ___ Rapid respiration
___ Coughing   ___ Other _____
___ Congestion   _____

Recommendation: _____

Figure 27-3 cont'd

Examination Checklist continued

Gastrointestinal System
___ Appears normal   ___ Abnormal feces
___ Excess gas   ___ Parasites
___ Vomiting   ___ Other _____
___ Anorexia   _____

Recommendation: _____

Urogenital System
___ Appears normal   ___ Enlarged prostate
___ Abnormal urination   ___ Mammary tumors
___ Genital discharge   ___ Other _____
___ Abnormal testicles   _____

Recommendation: _____

Anal Sacs
___ Appear normal   ___ Abscessed
___ Excessive fullness   ___ Other _____
___ Infected   _____
Recommendation: _____

Vaccination Schedule
___ Up to date
Due:
        ___ PARVO ___ Rabies   ___ FP ___ Other
Given:
        ___ PARVO ___ Rabies   ___ FP ___ Other

Figure 27-3 cont'd

Drawing Conclusions

1. Describe any abnormal findings from the assessment. What might be the cause of the abnormality, if one is found?

   _____

   _____

   _____

Critical Thinking

Animal Rights

Most scientists believe that research using animals is necessary to develop new treatments and drugs and to understand human behavior. Some people who care about the welfare of animals believe that research could be completed without using animals. The controversy also involves the use of animals for making fur coats and for testing cosmetics. More than 90% of the animals used in research are bred for that purpose.

Guidelines for laboratories that use animals in research have been developed by the National Institutes of Health (NIH). The laboratory must provide the NIH with written documentation to show the designs of the experiments. It must also document other work in the same field to show that the tests are not a duplication. The laboratory administration must pledge that animals used for research will not experience unnecessary pain without anesthesia.

Examining the Evidence

1. Which animal health care professional might be the best person to determine what is considered to be "humane care"? Explain your answer.

   _____

   _____

   _____

2. Why do you support or not support the use of animals for research purposes?

   _____

   _____

   _____

3. Why do or do you not believe that the guidelines used by the NIH to regulate research laboratories are adequate?

   _____

   _____

   _____

Prove It!

Animals have been attributed many benefits as pets. Some of these benefits include the ability to lower blood pressure, to protect, or to assist with activities of daily living. The manner in which people treat their pets has also been a subject of research. For example, some people treat their pet as a member of the family, buying presents, preparing and feeding them table food, and so forth. Another area of interest is the manner in which people speak to pets. Some address their pets with gestures as much or more than words, others are authoritative, and others speak in "baby talk."

Use the information above for ideas to design an experiment that will determine a characteristic of the relationship between people and their pets. Conduct the experiment and report the results to the class.

Examining the Evidence

1. What is the hypothesis of your experiment?

   _____

   _____

   _____

2. Describe the design of your experiment including materials and time limits.

_____

_____

_____

3. What is the controlled variable in your experiment?

_____

_____

_____

4. What is the variable in your experiment?

_____

_____

_____

5. What conclusion were you able to draw regarding your hypothesis?

_____

_____

_____

28 Community and Social Careers

Vapid Vocabulary

Before reading the chapter, review the glossary terms from the chapter in the word search puzzle below. Define each of the terms in the space provided.

```
N  O  I  T  N  E  V  R  E  T  N  I  B  V  A  E  D  O  N  I
E  N  A  A  T  M  E  O  T  C  N  A  E  A  T  N  T  N  C  E
N  T  C  T  R  N  Y  O  I  N  C  D  E  S  C  T  T  A  A  F
D  D  T  A  N  S  E  O  O  C  N  N  E  I  I  E  N  D  N  M
B  C  R  N  O  T  D  N  A  C  N  N  C  C  O  C  T  D  A  F
T  D  C  I  N  N  O  L  R  T  A  E  C  D  V  N  I  I  C  C
E  D  T  F  V  N  A  T  N  E  M  E  N  I  F  N  O  C  A  E
I  Y  C  N  E  U  Q  I  L  E  D  O  D  D  C  I  T  T  B  C
D  I  V  N  R  C  I  T  D  M  I  N  E  A  O  D  T  I  D  N
D  I  C  E  A  C  N  F  T  E  I  E  E  Y  G  C  A  O  T  O
E  A  A  C  A  O  I  T  U  E  A  N  N  G  N  T  R  N  A  T
C  T  C  I  A  I  D  M  C  D  I  O  I  D  I  E  Q  C  N  R
E  T  T  I  N  C  I  C  O  E  A  C  O  T  I  E  C  O  C
I  O  M  S  E  R  N  C  O  O  A  E  N  A  I  C  D  D  D  T
N  E  T  I  T  D  O  E  O  N  N  I  D  M  V  C  T  N  C  D
N  R  C  T  A  I  D  S  N  T  I  N  T  T  E  N  I  N  D  R
M  C  T  A  T  I  A  L  C  N  I  C  N  V  O  I  N  N  N  N
N  N  T  T  O  E  E  D  N  A  I  B  G  C  N  C  C  N  T  O
T  N  N  S  T  O  L  E  R  A  N  C  E  E  C  R  N  I  N  C
C  A  C  I  R  E  R  I  O  Y  C  A  C  O  V  D  A  N  A  R
```

1. Addiction- _____

2. Advocacy- _____

3. Baccalaureate- _____

4. Cognitive- _____

5. Confinement- _____

6. Gender- _____

7. Intervention- _____

8. Statistic- _____

9. Tolerance- _____

Key Search

Find the key terms of the chapter by matching the terms to the definitions in the space provided.

Term Tank	
Communicable .	Immunization
Demographic	Pollution
Dependence	Vector
Hallucination	Withdrawal

DEFINITION	KEY TERM
Pertaining to the study of people as a group, especially of statistical groupings according to age, gender, and environmental factors	
Unpleasant symptoms resulting with stoppage of drugs or substances on which a person is dependent; symptoms include anxiety, insomnia, irritability, impaired attention, and physical illness	
Capable of being transmitted from one person or animal to another	
Process of becoming secure against a particular disease or pathogen	
Carrier that transfers an infective agent from one host to another	
Sensory perception that occurs in waking state but does not have external stimulus	
Condition of being defiled or impure	
Addiction to drugs or alcohol	

Just the Facts

1. Community and social health care has broad goals and focuses on the health needs of a

   _ _ _ _ _ _ _ Ⓞ _ _.

2. The community and social health care Ⓞ_ _ _ _ _ is involved in the search for the

   source of _ _ _ _ _ _ _ and the use of technical and regulatory means to protect the

   population from environmental, social, and behavioral hazards

3. _ _ _ _ Ⓞ_ _ _ _ _ _ _ _ _ _ _ _ _ identify and explain

   the social factors affecting the care of patients.

4. _ _ _ _ _ _ _ _ _ _ _ _ _ _ _ Ⓞ_ _ _ _ _ _

   specialize in providing assistance to the elderly.

5. There are three levels of education for professional social workers including the bachelor's

   degree, the master's degree, and the _ _ _ _ _ _ _ _ degree.

6. _ _ _ _ _ _ _ _ _ _ help their patients to solve problems of personal, social,

   career, and educational development.

7. The _ _ _ _ _ _ _ _ _ _ _ _ _ _ _ Ⓞ_ _ _ _ works in

   health care settings and focuses on the emotional and developmental needs of children.

8. Drug dependence is the _ Ⓞ_ _ _ _ _ _ or

   _ _ _ _ _ _ _ _ _ _ _ _ Ⓞ_ need to continue taking a drug.

9. _ _ _ _ _ _ Ⓞ_ _ _ _ _ may be used to increase the activity of the central ner-

   vous system whereas Ⓞ_ _ _ _ _ _ _ _ _ _ _ have the opposite effect.

10. Two drugs that are commonly associated with _ _ _ _ Ⓞ_ _ _ are flunitrazepam

    and gamma hydroxybutrate.

Use the circled letters to form the answer to this jumble. Clue: What is the physical reaction to stopping a drug that has caused dependence called?

_ _ _ _ _ _ _ _ _ _

Concept Applications

Community and Social Health Careers

Community and Social Health Skills and Qualities

List three personal qualities and skills that are important in community and social health careers.

1. _____

2. _____

3. _____

Identifying Community and Social Health Careers

Use the textbook to complete the missing information about community and social health careers in Table 28-1.

TABLE 28-1

Career Title	Years of Education	Description of Job Duties and Opportunities	Credentials Required
			MS; most states require licensure
		Determine suitability of foster homes and adoption applicants	
		Provide daily care for children in institutions under supervision	
		Complete application for unemployment, food stamps and other services	
			BSW, MSW, DSW, ACSW

Applying Your Knowledge

1. The health practitioner who assists children who are confined in the hospital with play therapy may be educated as a _____.

2. Counselors who specialize in career opportunities and learning a trade are called

   _____.

3. A disabled child might be assisted while attending school by the _____.

4. Schools, rehabilitation agencies, mental health or correctional facilities, and colleges are just a few of the settings in which _____ work.

5. Counselors who specialize in substance abuse may be educated as _____ or

   _____.

Investigations

Observing the Spread of Microorganisms

Work in groups of six or seven people for this activity. Read all of the directions before beginning this activity. Laboratory activities should be completed only under the supervision of a qualified professional.

Equipment and Supplies

6 to 8 applicators
autoclave or bleach
beaker of warm water
grease pencil or china marker
incubator
package of dry yeast
1 peppermint candy
3 potato dextrose agar plates per group

Directions

1. Practice good medical asepsis by using frequent handwashing technique.

2. Use the skills listed in the textbook to prepare a sterile plate of potato dextrose agar.

3. Use a grease pencil to draw a line on the outside of each plate to divide the agar plate into halves or fourths as directed by the instructor. There should be one section of the plate for each student in the group.

4. Number each section of the plate consecutively to eight with the grease pencil.

5. Prepare a solution of warm water and baking yeast in a beaker.

6. Soak a piece of hard peppermint candy in the beaker for 3 to 5 minutes.

7. While the candy is soaking, all students of the group should wash their hands thoroughly with warm water and soap. Rinse completely.

8. Designate each student of the group with a number to correspond to the agar plate sections.

9. Student #1 should remove the candy from the beaker and rub it in the palm of his/her right hand. Discard the candy in an appropriate waste receptacle.

10. Student #1 shakes hands with student #2. Participants should not touch any surface with their hands after shaking hands with the previous student of the group until the culture is taken from the hand.

11. Student #2 shakes hands with student #3.

12. Student #3 shakes hands with student #4, and so forth to student #6 or #7. It is important that the handshaking be done rapidly down the line of students.

13. During the process of hand shaking, the last student should "culture" the palm of student #1 and streak section #1 of the plate with the specimen gathered. Student #1 may then wash his or her hands.

14. After student #1's culture is done, that student may culture student #2's palm and streak the section labeled #2 with the specimen.

15. After student #2's culture is done, the hands may be washed and that student may culture student #3's palm and streak the plate.

16. The procedure is continued until all students' palms have been cultured and plates have been streaked for each.

17. After the culturing is done, incubate the plates upside down at approximately 37° C for 24 hours. Observe the plates and record any growth that occurs.

18. Continue incubation and observation every day for 5 days.

19. Sterilize or disinfect the agar plates before discarding.

Drawing Conclusions

1. What type of organism was cultured on the potato dextrose agar? Did any other organism grow on the plates?

_____

_____

_____

2. In which section did growth occur first?

_____

_____

_____

3. In which section was the growth the heaviest?

_____

_____

_____

4. In which section was the growth the lightest?

_____

_____

_____

5. How was the organism transferred from student #1 to student #7?

_____

_____

_____

6. Why were all of the students' hands washed before the activity was started?

_____

_____

_____

7. Why didn't the plates contain growth of many types of organisms?

_____

_____

_____

8. Why is 37° C used for incubation of microorganisms?

_____

_____

_____

Critical Thinking

Unsolved Mysteries

This activity is adapted from the VQI (Vector Quest I) series developed by the Iowa Medical Foundation. It allows you to be an epidemiologist, or medical detective. Use the information to answer the questions.

Situation #1

Farmington, Iowa, is experiencing an increased rate of cancer cases and a resulting increase in deaths. The residents speculate about the power lines, old tanneries, the water, the air, and genetics. There could be any number of reasons including chance that would explain this cluster.

Examining the Evidence

1. What are the variables that might be considered in determining a solution to this mystery?

_____

_____

_____

2. What questions would you like answered to help you to determine the source of this cluster of illnesses?

_____

_____

_____

3. Describe how information could be obtained or an experiment performed to determine the source of this cluster.

_____

_____

_____

4. Are there any health measures that might be recommended to the the population of Farmington to limit the risk of developing this cancer?

_____

_____

_____

Situation #2

In the Northwest, Alaska Airlines has identified a particular plane that has a history of "making people sick."

Examining the Evidence

1. What are the variables that might be considered in determining a solution to this mystery?

   _____

   _____

   _____

2. What questions would you like answered to help you to determine the source of this cluster of illnesses?

   _____

   _____

   _____

3. Describe how information could be obtained or an experiment performed to determine the source of this cluster.

   _____

   _____

   _____

4. Are there any health measures that might be recommended to the airline to limit the risk of developing this disease?

   _____

   _____

   _____

29 Mental Health Careers

Vapid Vocabulary

Before reading the chapter, review the glossary terms from the chapter in the word search puzzle below. Define each of the terms in the space provided.

E	E	A	R	P	I	P	N	E	P	I	P	C	L	I	Y	Y	N	T	Y
E	N	T	N	T	R	D	R	F	S	E	N	N	L	U	N	P	U	N	E
R	P	E	Y	F	E	P	O	A	R	Y	Y	R	I	E	Y	I	T	E
P	S	R	I	Y	I	R	H	S	E	S	E	O	E	R	T	R	N	S	T
F	E	Y	A	G	E	L	E	V	I	T	A	T	I	T	N	A	U	Q	U
E	N	R	E	N	Y	V	A	F	O	S	O	P	T	I	M	A	L	N	I
S	F	I	S	A	E	H	N	N	F	I	S	E	R	O	Q	E	N	I	A
I	E	I	E	R	I	A	I	O	O	N	O	E	O	L	S	S	E	E	C
A	C	U	A	F	C	L	I	P	I	I	F	R	N	A	I	O	N	L	S
S	P	N	P	Y	N	F	F	N	O	S	T	T	N	Y	E	N	R	H	V
F	C	T	G	R	E	Q	N	U	E	I	N	C	E	U	E	A	H	C	O
E	P	N	I	P	O	S	T	V	E	R	D	P	N	F	E	N	E	N	I
Q	O	A	P	T	V	N	S	N	N	E	H	F	N	U	P	R	N	R	I
E	F	C	L	C	U	O	P	I	N	P	P	U	S	F	N	A	P	H
O	R	E	U	D	I	D	A	I	O	N	I	I	O	H	T	S	P	E	P
T	P	S	E	S	G	I	E	P	R	S	Y	N	O	Z	R	U	Z	O	A
F	P	R	R	I	S	N	Y	I	P	N	E	R	T	O	I	P	G	S	U
I	R	T	A	E	A	N	O	P	E	I	O	N	E	C	N	H	S	E	P
E	A	I	A	I	I	R	E	O	Y	G	E	I	R	E	E	T	C	P	S
P	E	S	N	T	E	E	I	U	F	N	N	R	Y	T	N	N	T	S	E

1. Aptitude- _____

2. Forensics- _____

3. Frayed- _____

4. Functional- _____

5. Inspire- _____

6. Hygiene- _____

7. Optimal- _____

8. Perseverance-_____

9. Quantitative- _____

10. Schizophrenia-_____

Key Search

Find the Key Terms of the chapter by matching the terms to the definitions in the space provided.

Term Tank	
Behavior	Psychosis
Phobia	Psychotherapy
Psychology	Reality orientation
Psychoneurosis	Restraint

DEFINITION	KEY TERM
Study of human and animal behavior, normal and abnormal	
Physical confinement	
Persistent abnormal dread or fear	
Conduct, actions that can be observed	
Treatment of discomfort, dysfunction, or diseases by methods designed to understand and cope with problems	
Awareness of position in relation to time, space, and person	
Functional disturbance of the mind in which the individual is aware that reactions are not normal	
Major mental disorder in which the individual loses contact with reality	

Just the Facts

1. The function of the mental health care team is to provide care and treatment for individuals with disorders of the _ _ _ ◯ , _ _ _ _ _ _ _ _, or _ _ _ _ _ _ _ _ ◯ .

2. It is now commonly accepted that a person's emotional and mental state may either cause or have some effect on all _ _ _ _ _ ◯ _ _ disorders.

3. _ _ _ _ _ _ ◯ _ _ _ _ _ _ are licensed physicians specializing in the treatment of mental, emotional, and behavioral disorders.

4. _ _ _ _ _ _ ◯ _ _ _ _ _ _ are professionals, not physicians, who specialize in treatment of mental and emotional disorders.

5. _ _ _ _ _ _ _ _ _ _ _ _ is a state of mind in which a person can cope with problems and maintain emotional balance and satisfaction in living.

6. _ _ _ _ _ _ ◯ _ _ _ _ _ _ _ are functional disturbances of the mind.

7. _ _ _ _ _ _ _ _ _ are severe or major mental disorders in which the individual is not in contact with reality.

8. Mental _ _ _ _ ◯ _ _ includes the methods used to preserve and promote mental health.

9. Loss of _ _ _ _ _ _ _ _ _ _ may result from loss of hearing, sight, or confinement.

10. Use of _ _ _ _ _ ◯ _ _ _ _ must be ordered by a physician and only after proper instruction is given for their use.

Use the circled letters to form the answer to this jumble. Clue: What is a useful tool in helping a patient maintain reality orientation?

_ _ _ _ _ _ _ _

Concept Applications

Recognizing Substance Abuse

List 10 signs and symptoms that might indicate substance abuse.

1. _____
   _____

2. _____
   _____

3. _____
   _____

4. _____
   _____

5. _____
   _____

6. _____
   _____

7. _____
   _____

8. _____
   _____

9. _____
   _____

10. _____
    _____

Applying Your Knowledge

1. Which of the signs and symptoms you have listed might result from causes other than substance abuse?

   _____
   _____
   _____

2. What type of intervention could you use with a person showing the signs and symptoms you have listed to determine if substance abuse is the cause?

   _____
   _____
   _____

3. What would you do if you were concerned that a friend might be using mind-altering substances?

_____

_____

_____

4. What resources are available in the community to help an individual with substance abuse problems?

_____

_____

_____

Identifying Mental Messages

Psychosocial health care professionals often use the concept of "self-talk" in helping people deal with emotional concerns. Each person receives many positive and negative messages from others and themselves every day. Complete Table 29-1 by changing the negative message to one that is positive. Add five negative messages that you give to yourself or someone else gives you. Change the negative message into one that is positive.

TABLE 29-1

	Message–Negative	Message–Positive
Example	I am (you are) always late.	I have a tendency to be late, but through better planning I can arrive on time.
	I (you) can't ever get a B in math.	_____
		_____
	I'm (you're) so fat.	_____
		_____
	I (you) never get along with him/her.	_____
		_____
	I'm (you're) such a slob.	_____
		_____
	_____	_____
	_____	_____
	_____	_____
	_____	_____

Mental Health Careers

Mental Health Skills and Qualities

List three personal qualities and skills that are important in mental health careers.

1. _____

2. _____

3. _____

Identifying Mental Health Careers

Use the textbook to complete the missing information about mental health careers in Table 29-2.

TABLE 29-2

Career Title	Years of Education	Description of Job Duties and Opportunities	Credentials Required
			PhD, EdD, or PsyD
		Interview, lead group sessions, give daily care, make home visits, in some states may administer medications	
		Treatment of mental, emotional and behavioral disorders; may prescribe medications	
	4- to 6-month program or on-the-job training		

Applying Your Knowledge

1. For treatment of a mental disorder that requires medication, the client would probably seek the care of a _____.

2. Assistance with activities of daily living such as reality orientation would probably be accomplished by the _____ working under the supervision of the professional.

3. In some state the health care worker called the _____ is also called a mental health associate or human service worker..

4. The professional who uses interviews, testing, and observation to treat mental disorders but does not prescribe medication is called a _____.

5. The mental health specialist who practices in diverse areas of cllinical, quantitative, consumer, environmental, and organizational behavior is probably a _____.

Critical Thinking

Mental Health Stigma

Most people who suffer from mental disorders recover completely and live active and productive lives. Understanding and treatment of the mentally ill has evolved from placing the individual with a mental disorder in an asylum to allowing the person active participation in society.

However, a stigma (or attitude) still exists in society that people with mental disorders are weak or violent. Some people believe that all mentally ill people should be "locked up" and kept away from others.

In the 1970s a man was considered by a political party to run for vice president of the United States. The man led an active and complete life. He had a family and had done many great things in his community and political party. However, when it became known that he had been treated at one time for a mental disorder, the party dropped his name from the ticket.

Examining the Evidence

1. Why do some people believe that people with mental illnesses are weak or violent?

   _____

   _____

   _____

2. When should limitations be placed on the activities of a person with a mental disorder?

   _____

   _____

   _____

3. For what kind of disorder to you believe that a mentally ill person should be refused a driver's license?

   _____

   _____

   _____

4. How might the political party's decision to drop the candidate from their ticket affect another person who is suffering from depression or other mental disorders but wants to run for political office in the future?

   _____

   _____

   _____

What's "News"?

In 1994, research studies reported results of studies regarding human psychosocial behavior, some of which were controversial. Respond to each of the following conclusions that researchers drew from their studies. Use examples from your own experiences or information you have learned to agree or disagree with the research.

Psychologists reported that memories of stressful and emotional events are retained longer due to release of hormones.

Response:

_____

_____

_____

In a study using rhesus monkeys, it was determined that certain behaviors keep aggression in control in crowded conditions.

Response:

_____

_____

_____

Researchers determined that babies babble with acoustic structure and patterns of speech at 2 months of age. Others concluded that babies recognize their name at 4.5 months of age.

Response:

_____

_____

_____

30 Rehabilitative Careers

Vapid Vocabulary

Before reading the chapter, review the glossary terms from the chapter in the word search puzzle below. Define each of the terms in the space provided.

```
D  I  F  I  C  A  I  L  T  C  N  S  P  G  O  C  E  N  P  T
I  F  U  A  S  H  S  E  A  F  I  I  L  B  R  N  O  E  U  H
S  T  O  E  N  T  A  S  L  T  N  T  I  C  N  N  R  E  C  S
C  H  L  N  S  N  L  C  A  I  I  E  Y  C  E  C  O  C  F  A
R  O  O  C  N  I  I  N  M  T  A  N  C  L  U  L  T  C  F  A
I  R  O  E  O  C  O  N  I  F  I  C  E  S  A  I  I  N  L  T
M  T  O  E  C  U  C  O  N  O  O  O  S  G  N  N  T  T  C  I
I  I  A  I  L  T  I  I  A  F  N  I  N  N  N  I  A  A  O  S
N  C  N  I  Y  O  A  T  R  G  O  I  A  I  O  O  O  C  O  N
A  U  L  V  O  A  G  A  A  N  F  A  I  A  O  N  C  S  N  C
T  L  S  C  O  N  S  C  I  E  N  T  I  O  U  S  R  E  E  G
I  T  T  O  I  T  S  I  R  S  S  N  F  E  O  R  A  N  M  O
O  U  N  N  F  A  R  F  T  T  I  I  I  T  L  A  T  R  R
N  R  H  L  V  S  L  B  L  N  S  R  E  O  I  A  A  R  F  F
T  A  A  Y  N  I  I  A  O  C  R  N  C  W  O  O  T  T  M  O
O  L  I  A  T  N  L  F  W  N  A  F  O  I  N  N  H  O  F  I
C  I  S  F  O  T  A  O  Y  N  I  N  I  S  C  L  R  O  O  O
E  L  L  I  A  R  B  N  T  R  R  E  L  I  O  N  I  H  C  C
O  E  O  C  U  N  L  L  U  I  N  C  E  N  T  I  V  E  I
O  C  N  N  O  N  O  S  A  N  Y  H  I  N  E  N  L  I  O  I
```

1. Analytic- _____

2. Braille- _____

3. Congenital- _____

4. Conscientious- _____

5. Discrimination- _____

6. Fabrication- _____

7. Horticultural- _____

8. Incentive-_____

9. Laminar airflow- _____

10. Percussion- _____

Key Search

Find the Key Terms of the chapter by matching the terms to the definitions in the space provided.

Term Tank			
Articulation	Dosage	Orthotics	Rehabilitation
Audiology	Frequency	Pharmacology	Therapy
Disability	Hydrotherapy	Prosthesis	
Dispense	Nebulizer	Prosthetics	

DEFINITION	KEY TERM
Regulation of size, frequency, and amount of medication	
Number of times an event occurs in a given period	
Art or science of custom designing, fabrication, and fitting of braces	
Artificial device applied to replace a partially or totally missing body part	
Study of the actions and uses of drugs	
Enunciation of words and syllables, how sounds are spoken	
Treatment of disease; science and art of healing	
Science of hearing	
Prepare, package, compound, or label for delivery according to a lawful order of a qualified practitioner	
Restoration of normal form and funciton after injury or illness	

Term Tank continued on following page

Term Tank continued from following page

DEFINITION	KEY TERM
Art or science of custom design, fabrication, and fitting of artificial limbs	
Device used to deliver a spray or mist of medication into the lungs	
Lack of ability to function in the manner that most people function physically or mentally	
Application of water	

Just the Facts

1. The _ _ _ _ _ _ _ _ _ _ _ _ _ _ ◯ team provides services designed to overcome physical, developmental, behavioral, or emotional disabilities.

2. _ _ _ _ _ _ _ ◯ _ therapists work to restore function, relieve pain, and prevent _ _ _ _ _ _ _ _ _ _ _ after disease, injury, or loss of a body part.

3. _ _ ◯ _ _ _ _ _ _ _ _ _ _ _ _ _ _ _ _ help patients strengthen and coordinate body movements using exercise.

4. _ _ _ _ _ _ _ _ _ _ _ _ modify and provide footwear to patients with imperfectly formed feet.

5. _ _ _ ◯ _ _ _ _ _ _ ◯ _ therapy helps patients reach the highest level of independent living by overcoming physical injury, birth defects, aging, or emotional and developmental problems.

6. _ _ _ ◯ _ _ _ _ _ _ _ _ _ ◯ _ _ _ work under the supervision of the team physician in a variety of amateur and professional sports and other settings.

7. _ _ _ _ _ _ _ _ _ _ _ ◯ mix and dispense drugs according to prescriptions written by physicians, veterinarians, dentists, and other authorized professionals.

8. _ _ _ _ _ _ _ ◯ _ _ _ _ therapists evaluate the patient to administer respiratory care and operate life support equipment under the supervision of a physician

9. _ _ _ _ _ _ _ _ _ ◯ _ _ _ is the study of drugs, their actions, dosages, side effects, indications, and contraindications.

10. _ _ Ⓞ _ and Ⓞ _ _ _ applications are used in physical therapy to allow increased movement of joints.

Use the circled letters to form the answer to this jumble. Clue: What is one of three common methods used to administer oxygen?

_ _ _ _ _   _ _ _ _ _ _ _

Concept Applications

Comparing Fluid Measurements

Three systems are currently used to measure fluid volumes: the SI (or metric), apothecary, and household systems. The metric system was developed in France, is used internationally, and is based on the decimal system using units of 10. The apothecary system was the original system used in the United States by pharmacists. The household system was developed for use with common items found in the home. Study the chart of approximate equivalents to answer the questions.

METRIC	APOTHECARY	HOUSEHOLD
1000 mL	32 oz	1 qt
500 mL	16 oz	1 pt
30 mL	1 oz	2 T
4 mL	1 dr	1 tsp
0.06 mL	1 min	1 gt

KEY TO SYMBOLS
cc = cubic centimeter
mL = mL
oz = fluid ounce (f℥)
dr = fluid dram (f℈)
min = fluid minim (℔)
qt = quart
pt = pint
T = tablespoon
tsp = teaspoon
gt = drop

Applying Your Knowledge

1. How many ounces are equivalent to 60 cc?

   _____

   _____

   _____

2. How many drops are equivalent to 1 teaspoon?

   _____

   _____

   _____

3. How many cubic centimeters are equivalent to 10 ounces?

_____

_____

_____

4. How many liters are equivalent to 1200 cc?

_____

_____

_____

5. Which system is most easily changed from one unit of measurement to another in the same system?

_____

_____

_____

Calculating Drug Dosages

Use Figure 30-1 in the textbook to calculate the dosage problems.

Applying Your Knowledge

1. The order is to give the client a medication at the dosage of 10 mL every hour. What would the correct dosage be in teaspoons?

_____

_____

_____

2. The order is to give the client a medication at the dosage of 300 mg. You have tablets that are 500 mg strength. How many tablets would you need to give the client for a correct dosage?

_____

_____

_____

3. The order is to give the client a medication at the dosage of 15 mg/kg of weight, three times a day. You have a dosage of grains. The client weighs 120 pounds. How much of the medicaiton do you need to have on hand for a 24-hour period?

_____

_____

_____

Using the Manual Alphabet

Use Figure 30-5 in the textbook to decode the message in Figure 30-1. Construct a message of your own. Practice "signing" the message with a partner.

Careers in 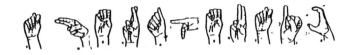 health

provide the 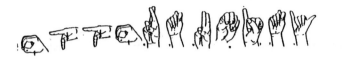 to

work with 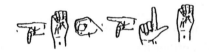 who have emotional,

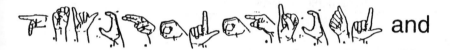 and

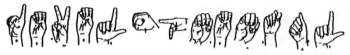 problems.

Figure 30-1

Applying Your Knowledge

1. What does the message say?

   _____

   _____

   _____

2. Why would it be preferable to some hearing-impaired individuals to use signs that indicate words rather than letters?

   _____

   _____

   _____

3. Approximately 10% of the parents of hearing-impaired individuals learn to sign. Why might this be true?

   _____

   _____

   _____

Rehabilitative Careers

Rehabilitative Skills and Qualities

List three personal qualities and skills that are important in rehabilitative careers.

1. _____

2. _____

3. _____

Identifying Rehabiliative Careers

Use the textbook to complete the missing information about rehabilitative careers in Table 30-2.

TABLE 30-1

Career Title	Years of Education	Description of Job Duties and Opportunities	Credentials Required
		Design, fabricate, and fit braces and strengthening devices	
	1800-hour internship		
			BS; MS preferred; licensed by the state
		Analyze activities to provide assistance to disabled people to accomplish activities of daily living; plan and supervise programs	
			PharmD or BS Pharm

Applying Your Knowledge

1. One of the therapeutic careers that is a form of psychotherapy and involves movement is called

   _____.

2. Artificial kidneys are run by practitioners called _____, and this career may be learned _____.

3. Language problems may be diagnosed by the _____ whereas hearing problems are directed to the _____.

4. Oxygen administration and the use of breathing treatments such as incentive spirometry are skills performed by the _____.

5. During surgery and respiratory failure, the patient's heart and lungs may be replaced by a machine run by the _____.

Critical Thinking

Care of Hearing Aids

Hearing aids are devices that act as miniature loudspeakers to make sounds louder. The hearing aid does not cure the hearing impairment. It requires proper care and maintenance to be effective. Hearing aids may be worn:

- In the ear
- Behind the ear
- Behind the ear with a plastic tube leading into the ear canal
- Built into eyeglasses
- Clipped to the wearer's clothing with a cord and button like receiver in the ear

The following are simple guidelines to use when speaking to an individual wearing a hearing aid and steps for care of the hearing aid:

1. Face the person directly when speaking.
2. Speak clearly, slowly, and naturally.
3. Do not place the hearing aid in direct sunlight or on hot surfaces.
4. Do not use hair sprays while the hearing aid is in place.
5. Do not get the hearing aid wet.
6. Clean the ear mold by carefully removing wax with a pipe cleaner or toothpick.
7. Wash the ear mold in mild soap and water if it can be detached from the hearing aid.
8. Inspect the tubing for cracks, loose connections, and twisting, which may indicate the need for relacement.

Examining the Evidence

1. Would it be necessary to speak loudly to a person wearing a hearing aid?

   _____

   _____

   _____

2. Why is it important to remove the hearing aid before taking a shower or bath?

   _____

   _____

   _____

3. Rubbing alcohol has the property of drying materials. Why is it important to avoid the use of it when cleaning hearing aids?

   _____

   _____

   _____

Living with Disabilities

Physical disabilities affect people of every age, race, and socioeconomic status. It is estimated that up to 40 million Americans have some form of physical disability. These disabilities may be the result of stroke, head or spinal injury, arthritis, neurologic disease, or back pain. The following questions are designed to help you explore your knowledge and attitude about disabilities.

Examining the Evidence

1. What are three adaptations that have been made for students who use a wheelchair in your school?

   _____

   _____

   _____

2. Are there any areas of your school that are inaccessible to students in a wheelchair?

   _____

   _____

   _____

3. What are three adaptive techniques that would be needed when caring for a person without sight?

   _____

   _____

   _____

4. Do you think that a disabled person would appreciate being looked at or away from when you are walking past?

   _____

   _____

   _____

5. Do you think that it is a good idea to talk to a disabled person about the disability or to avoid talking about the disability?

   _____

   _____

   _____

6. Do you think that a person with limited mobility would appreciate or resent help with tasks, such as putting on a coat or lifting books?

   _____

   _____

   _____

31 *Emergency Health Careers*

Vapid Vocabulary

Before reading the chapter, review the glossary terms from the chapter in the word search puzzle below. Define each of the terms in the space provided.

```
L A T I N E G E H L E U E D I N M I A L
L O A T E E M U E R R R E M O L E L E N
L H G I L B U S I L R F E R E H D A E L
E H A N O O T B A D I E I A U I I A R A
A L A L U L E A E B N C U U P R R A T E
E E I N Y I N M R M D S L L E R E E T M
Y S L S L C C I T C A L Y H P A N A R R
M R E B R L L M U E L O R T E P L E E B
N Y A E I L N B P R B L E E I N L N T C
E I L H A T T R E A S U A M N E E T T C
Y R M T N E P N A E A A D R E N A L I N
I L I I I M M E R S E C R U N A U I R R
A O G A R H P A C S R T L A N E B C T M
N L G R I R A C E S A U S A N N B E M L
A T L N E E O A R I U N L L N E A A U R
I A R E E E L T E L L S E E U E I G L A
L R L U R N R H M T C A I L N N P E A A
C R A S E G L R B D N S U R I D E A A E
A A G N E N E E R R A O E E U T P E E N
O U A A E A N N Y E B A A I A S Y A P I
```

1. Adhere- _____

2. Adrenalin- _____

3. Allergen- _____

4. Anaphylactic- _____

5. Defibrillation- _____

6. Embolism-_____

7. Genital- _____

8. Immerse-_____

9. Petroleum-_____

10. Susceptible-_____

Key Search

Find the Key Terms of the chapter by matching the terms to the definitions in the space provided.

Term Tank

Aspiration	Critical	Resuscitation	Toxin
Aura	Endotracheal intubation	Seizure	
Cardiopulmonary	Hemorrhage	Shock	
Consciousness	Mottled	Tourniquet	

DEFINITION	KEY TERM
Instrument used to compress a blood vessel by application around an extremity	
Pertaining to the heart and lungs	
Condition of acute failure of the peripheral circulation	
Act of inhaling foreign matter, usually emesis, into the respiratory tract	
Abnormal external or internal bleeding	
Poison produced by animals, plants, or bacteria	
Restoration of life or consciousness of a person who is apparently dead by using artificial respiration and cardiac massage	
Subjective sensation or motor phenomenon that precedes and marks the onset of a seizure	
Sudden attack of a disease; uncontrolled muscle movements of epilepsy	
Responsiveness of the mind and to the impressions made by the senses	

DEFINITION	KEY TERM
Pertaining to a crisis or danger of death	
Placing a tube within or through the trachea	
Spotted, with patches of color	

Just the Facts

1. The goal of modern emergency care is immediate aid, or first aid, at the _ O _ _ _ _ _ _ _ _ _ _ _ _ _.

2. Emergency medical technicians work under the supervision of a O _ _ _ _ _ _ _ _ _ to provide care to the acutely ill or injured person in the prehospital setting.

3. The EMT–P, or _ _ _ _ _ _ _ _ _ _, provides advanced life support.

4. _ _ _ _ _ _ _ _ _ _ _ _ _ O professions have evolved as a career opportunity with the use of helicopters to transport victims to emergency facilities.

5. The first priority of the rescuer is to _ _ _ _ _ _ the victim from any immediate danger and determine the level of _ _ O _ _ _ _ _ _ _ _ _ _ _ of the victim.

6. _ _ _ _ _ _ is the response of the cardiovascular system to the presence of adrenaline resulting in capillary constriction.

7. The severity of a burn is determined by the _ _ _ _ O _ _ _ _, _ _ _ _ _ _, and _ _ _ _ _.

8. _ _ _ _ _ _ O _ _ _ _ can be classified as closed or open.

9. Exposure to heat can result in muscle _ _ _ _ _ _ _ _ _, heat _ _ _ _ O _ _ _ _ _, or _ _ _ _ _ _ _ _ _ _ _.

10. All emergency workers use substance isolation precautions to prevent the spread of _ _ _ O _ _ _ _ _ _ _ _ _ _.

Use the circled letters to form the answer to this jumble. Clue: What is one type of injury that has a high change of infection because the injury is not exposed to air?

_ _ _ _ _ _ _ _ _

Concept Applications

Identifying Pressure Points

Use Figure 31-8 in the textbook to label the pressure points in Figure 29-1.

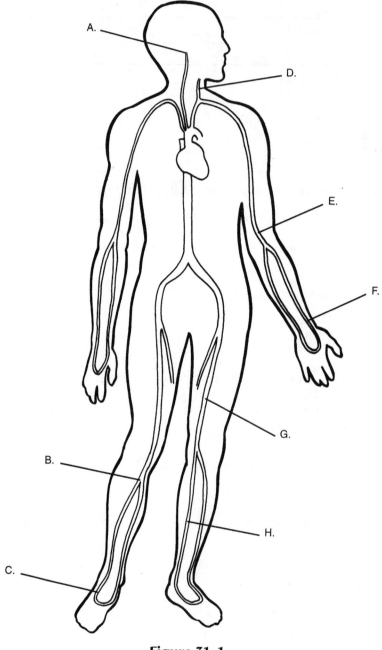

Figure 31-1

A. _____   **E.** _____

B. _____   **F.** _____

C. _____   **G.** _____

D. _____   **H.** _____

Inventing First Aid Reminders

Acronyms or sayings made by letters are often used to assist the memory. One acronym commonly used in first aid is "ABCs" to list the steps for assessment and the cardiopulmonary resuscitation (CPR) procedure. Choose one of the first aid situations from the textbook and design an acronym to help you remember the steps for care.

LETTER   ACTION STEP

_____ = _____

_____ = _____

_____ = _____

_____ = _____

_____ = _____

_____ = _____

_____ = _____

_____ = _____

_____ = _____

Applying Your Knowledge

1. What are the actions steps for the acronym "ABC"?

   _____

   _____

   _____

2. Name one other acronym that you have used to remember an action plan.

   _____

   _____

   _____

Emergency Careers

Emergency Skills and Qualities

List three personal qualities and skills that are important in emergency careers.

1. _____

2. _____

3. _____

Identifying Emergency Careers

Use the textbook to complete the missing information about emergency careers in Table 31-1.

TABLE 31-1

Career Title	Years of Education	Description of Job Duties and Opportunities	Credentials Required
			EMT–I; certification required
		Work in prehospital situation to provide care to victim of accident, injury, or illness; may administer medications and monitor electrocardiogram equipment	
			BSN, licensure required
	110 or more hours of supervised education		
			AHA and ARC offer classes for education

Investigations

Casualty Simulation

Read all of the directions before beginning this activity. Laboratory activities should be completed only under the supervision of a qualified professional.

Equipment and Supplies

newspaper
pillows
sheets

Directions

1. Choose a partner to role play one of the casualty simulations.

2. Choose a third person to act as the victim.

3. Consult with your partner for 3 minutes about the situation before beginning the role play.

4. Other members of the class may act as observers and evaluate the care given to the victim using Figure 31-2.

5. Switch roles to complete the simulations.

```
┌─────────────────────────────────────────────────────────────────────┐
│              EVALUATION SCALE FOR CASUALTY SIMULATION                 │
│                                                                       │
│    Communicates effectively with victim              ____ / 10 points │
│    Communicates effectively with partner             ____ / 5 points  │
│    Volunteers pertinent information about assessment                   │
│    and first aid treatment                           ____ / 5 points  │
│    Assesses victim for known and unknown injuries    ____ / 10 points │
│    Correctly treats injuries                         ____ / 10 points │
│    Gives first aid care quickly                      ____ / 5 points  │
│    Uses safety measures to protect victim and selves ____ / 5 points  │
│    TOTAL TEAM SCORE:                                 ____ / 50 points │
└─────────────────────────────────────────────────────────────────────┘
```

Figure 31-2

Casualty Simulation Victims

Situation One

Your victim was working on a power pole and touched a live wire while unsuccessfully trying to break a fall. The fall was approximately 20 feet. His right hand has a third-degree burn diagonally across the palm from the contact with the wire. There are also some first- and second-degree burns around the area of the third-degree burn. The victim is responsive and complaining of severe pain in his lower right arm.

Situation Two

Your victim was kicked in the chest by a horse. You find her sitting against a fencepost. She is dazed and confused but responsive. She is complaining of numbness and a tingling sensation in her left arm. You can see that the left arm is displaced in a downward direction from a break in the left clavicle.

Situation Three

Your victim was running up the bleachers at school and slipped. He fell down the bleachers to the concrete below. He has a compound fracture of the left femur with moderate bleeding. He is responsive and complains of difficulty breathing.

Situation Four

Your victim is a student in a chemistry class. He knocked over a gas burner and some flammable liquid chemicals. The burning liquid ignited his shirt and jeans. The teacher pushed the student under the shower and put out the fire with water. The victim has first- and second-degree burns on his chest and both upper legs. He is pacing around the room and screaming that the pain is unbearable.

Situation Five

Your victim was injured in a car accident. She has a fractured jaw and closed fracture of the right lower arm. She is responsive but confused.

Situation Six

Your victim had an accident while riding an all-terrain vehicle in the desert. You do not know how long the victim was in the desert after the accident. His breathing is rapid and shallow. His pulse rate is very fast. He is not responsive. His skin is hot and dry to the touch. A bruise is visible on his left upper arm and the bone looks out of place in that area.

Drawing Conclusions

1. What first aid consideration must be made for all of the victims?

   _____

   _____

   _____

2. For each of the emergency situations described, list one measure that might have been used to prevent the injury.

   SITUATION #1: _____

   _____

   _____

   _____

   SITUATION #2: _____

   _____

   _____

   SITUATION #3: _____

   _____

   _____

   _____

   SITUATION #4: _____

   _____

   _____

   _____

   SITUATION #5: _____

   _____

   _____

   _____

   SITUATION #6: _____

   _____

   _____

   _____

Critical Thinking

Understanding Survival

The headlines of the 1983 newspaper read, "Dead Tot Improving at Hospital." The article reported the story of a boy aged 2 years, who, wearing only pajamas, wandered from his home in subzero temperatures. He was found frozen in the snow hours later with a core body temperature of 60° F. He had no vital signs present, and all his extremities were frozen. Health care workers resuscitated the boy and slowly returned his body temperature to normal. Although he had some damaged tissue from the freezing, the boy suffered no heart or brain damage from the ordeal.

A Chicago boy fell through the ice while sledding by Lake Michigan in 1984 and was submerged under water for about 20 minutes. Doctors were able to bring the boy back to life by maintaining life support and placing him in a drug-induced coma while raising his body temperature to normal.

Examining the Evidence

1. What may have allowed these boys to live through "death" without apparent brain damage due to lack of oxygen?

   _____

   _____

   _____

2. What other injuries might occur as a result of the body tissues freezing?

   _____

   _____

   _____

3. How did the drug-induced coma help the boy in his recovery from the Chicago incident?

   _____

   _____

   _____

"RICE" is Nice

Athletic trainers work to provide sports enthusiasts with a safe and productive training schedule. They are also the primary emergency care givers when an injury is sustained by the athlete during practice or an athletic event. One acronym used by trainers to give immediate care for minor injuries to muscles, tendons, and ligaments is "RICE" or "ICE-R." After the initial assessment to rule out fractures, the athletic trainer wants to control bleeding, inflammation, muscle spasm, and pain resulting from the injury. "RICE" stands for Rest, Ice, Compression, and Elevation.

With RICE treatment, the activity is stopped if pain is severe. Ice is placed on the injured area for 15 to 20 minutes. An elastic wrap is placed around the area affected. The painful area is elevated above the heart when possible.

Examining the Evidence

1. Why is the "ice" part of RICE used for muscular injuries?

    _____

    _____

    _____

2. Why is the "compression" part of RICE used for muscular injuries?

    _____

    _____

    _____

3. Why is the "elevation" part of RICE used for muscular injuries?

    _____

    _____

    _____

4. Why is the "rest" part of RICE used for muscular injuries?

    _____

    _____

    _____

5. In addition to preventing further injury, describe one other goal that the athletic trainer would have in the treatment of a muscular injury.

    _____

    _____

    _____

32 Information and Administration Careers

Vapid Vocabulary

Before reading the chapter, review the glossary terms from the chapter in the word search puzzle below. Define each of the terms in the space provided.

```
N O I T A T I D E R C C A S T T R I E T
E V I T A I T I N I E T N U R I A N B R
L E N N O S R E P R R T E B A T T A T A
E T R A I I C R N N T V R O N O I V R A
A E N A T C B R B A I D T R S S A E I E
N G I R S A E A N T F C N D A T E B I B
I O E I T I C S I S I E N I C T V I U R
I O I I N T T A E C A E N T B E A R A
T E T T A A E N I A A T A A I T T T N C
I C T T A P I S U A T C E T O G S P R C
M I N I E R T T N U I N G E N A V C T T
A S I R I I T D Y R O T A L U B M A N T
I B R B Y B T S E E N E S N I V O N I O
I V T T E T A N I D R O O C T E R S T
B T R I S N E E T G C E N I C S N I Y E
C I S A B R R E I R E T T E T N T A O C
N R B I A E R A E E R E I A E E A N I
V A I T I I P T T E R E A U I E T I I B
E T C E A I T O I I A E B E T O E D D E
T A I R B Y A A B A I A T C T N T R E A
```

1. Accreditation-_____

2. Ambulatory-_____

3. Certification-_____

4. Coordinate-_____

5. Initiative-_____

6. Personnel-_____

7. Registration-_____

8. Repetitive-_____

9. Subordinate-_____

10. Transaction-_____

Key Search

Find the Key Terms of the chapter by matching the terms to the definitions in the space provided.

Term Tank		
Administration	Customary	Reasonable
Benefit	Deficiency	Transcribe
Chart	Dictation	
Confidential	Insurance	

DEFINITION	**KEY TERM**
Fee charged by similar practitioners for a service in the same economic and geographical area	
To make a written copy of dictated or recorded matter	
Management, performance of executive responsibilities and duties	
Payment by contract by one party to another in which the second party guarantees the first party against financial loss from a specific event	
Fee that considers both the usual fee charged by a practitioner for a particular service and the fee charged by other practitioners for the same service	
Financial help in time of illness, retirement, or unemployment	
Speaking words to be written by another person; may be recorded	

DEFINITION	KEY TERM
Collection of written materials relating to the health care of a patient	
Lacking some important part	
Private and secret; may be protected by law	

Just the Facts

1. Careers in _ _ _ _ _ _ _ _ _ _ _ _ _ _ _ include the health care facility managers, supervisors, medical secretaries, unit coordinators, and medical records personnel.

2. Administrators Ⓞ_ _ _ _ _ _ _ _ _ services, hiring, and training of personnel.

3. Patient representatives, or Ⓞ_ _ _ _ _ _ _ _ _, help patients to understand the health care policies and procedures of the facility, obtain services, and make informed decisions about their care.

4. The _ _ _ _ _ _ _ _ _ _ _ _ _Ⓞ_ _ _ is employed by institutions and private facilities, such as a doctor's office, to assist in administration of services.

5. The health unit coordinator (HUC) performs _ _ _ _ _ _ _ _ _ _ _ activities for the nursing unit.

6. Medical _ _ _ _ _ _ _ personnel organize, analyze, and generate data relating to patient records.

7. The medical _ _ _ _ _ _ _ _ _ _ _ _ _ _ _ _ listens to and types information to provide a permanent record from a variety of audio equipment.

8. Ⓞ_ provide access to information by practicing professionals, researchers, and students.

9. Orderliness of equipment and supplies used in the work area provides a secure environment for maintaining the _ _ _ _ _ _ _ _ _ _ _ _ _ _ _ of patient records.

10. Ⓞ_ _ _ _ _ _ _ must be accurate, legible, complete, and organized to provide efficient care.

Use the circled letters to form the answer to this jumble. Clue: What is the collection of papers, test results, and patient information called?

_ _ _ _ _

Concept Applications

Composing a Business Letter

On your own sheet of paper, type or print a letter using the following information. You work for a medical doctor as a front office assistant. You have noticed that the account of Mrs. Adrienne Jones is overdue. Insurance has paid for all of the expenses of her care except for $180 visit for a second opinion with an associate in the office. Your doctor asks you to write a letter to Mrs. Jones to remind her of the fee due. The doctor asks you to keep in mind as you are writing the letter that Mrs. Jones's husband of 50 years died 6 months ago and that she might not be familiar with billing and insurance procedures. Mrs. Jones's address is 2325 S. Wilshire Blvd., Anytown, USA, 00345. You may create your own doctor's name and address.

Applying Your Knowledge

1. Explain why you think that you should or should not mention the loss of Mrs. Jones's husband in the letter.

   _____

   _____

   _____

2. Design a standard form letter to indicate fees that are due so that only the name, address, service performed, and amount owed need to be added before mailing.

Keeping a Budget Ledger

Complete the following daily log of charges and receipts in Figure 32-1. Complete the receipt form in Figure 32-2 for client Dwight Nelson.

Applying Your Knowledge

1. What is the total of the payments for the day?

   _____

   _____

   _____

2. Which clients do not owe any money to date?

   _____

   _____

   _____

3. What is the total for checks received on the date shown?

   _____

   _____

   _____

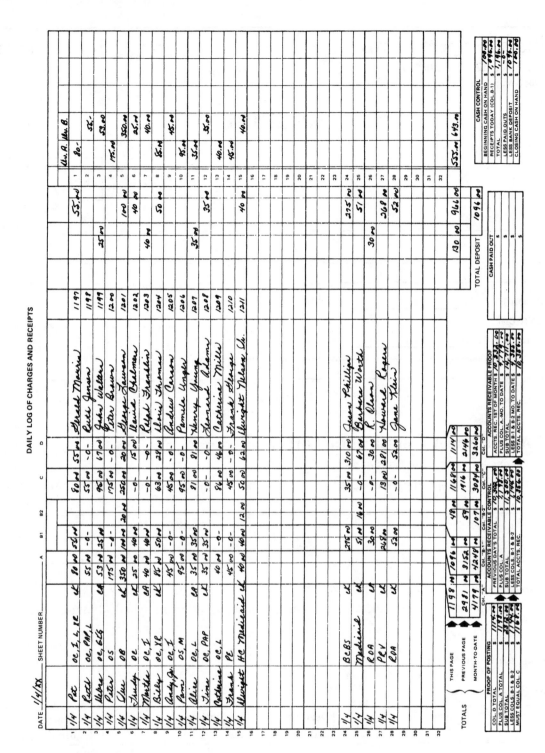

Figure 32-1 Daily ledger (From Cooper, Cooper, Burrows: *The Medical Assistant*, ed 6, St. Louis 1993, Mosby–Year Book, courtesy of Colwell Systems, Champaign, IL)

Clifford Temperson, MD
1023 Gentileer Drive, Suite 413
Anywhereville, Anystate, 12345

Date _____ 19 ___   No. 23100

RECEIPT

Received from

_____

$ _____

_____ Dollars

For _____

Account _____	___ Cash	Received by
Payment _____	___ Check	
Balance due _____	___ Money order	_____

Figure 32-2

Information and Administration Careers

Information and Administration Skills and Qualities

List three personal qualities and skills that are important in information and administration careers.

1. _____
2. _____
3. _____

Identifying Information and Administration Careers

Use the textbook to complete the missing information about information and administration careers in Table 32-1.

Applying Your Knowledge

TABLE 32-1

Career Title	Years of Education	Description of Job Duties and Opportunities	Credentials Required
			RRA
			CEO
		Perform duties of receptionist, accountant, and assistant; use telephone	
		Assist the patient to understand health care practices and policies	
			HUC

1. A patient might seek help with preparing a living will or resolving a conflict in the facility from the health care worker called a(n) _____.

2. The health care worker who listens to and prints audio recordings of information is called a(n) _____.

3. Access to printed information by health care professionals is often the responsibility of the _____.

4. Individuals who take photographs are often prepared with a _____ education.

5. Analyzing information relating to current trends in the health of a community is probably the responsibility of the _____.

Admitting a Patient

Directions

1. Choose partners to role play the admission of a patient to the facility using Figure 32-3.

2. Provide feedback to the person who is doing the admission about the clarity of instruction and manner.

3. Switch roles and complete the admission procedure again.

Date:_____ Time:_____ Introduced: Self_____ Roommate _____

Admitted per: Wheelchair_____ Cart _____ Ambulatory_____ Carried by _____

Age:_____ Sex: M _____ F _____

Condition on admission:

Ambulatory ☐	Feeds self ☐	Admitted by ambulance ☐	Alert ☐
Semiambulatory ☐	Requires help with feeding ☐	From hospital ☐	Forgetful ☐
Chairridden ☐	Continent ☐	From home ☐	Confused ☐
Bedridden ☐	Incontinent ☐	From nursing home ☐	

State of consciousness: Alert _____ Confused _____ Semiconscious _____ Unconscious _____

Emotional state: Calm _____ Nervous _____ Fearful _____ Angry _____ Depressed _____

Pain: No _____ Yes _____ Where _____

Vital signs: BP _____ T _____ P _____ R _____ Ht _____ Wt _____

Glasses: Yes_____ No _____ Contact lenses: Yes_____ No _____ Hearing aid: Yes_____ No_____

Dentures: Yes _____ No _____ Artificial limb: Yes _____ No_____

Artificial eye: Yes _____ No _____ Right _____ Left _____ Pacemaker: Yes _____ No _____

Orientation to environment:

Call light_____ Emergency light_____ Bed controls_____ Bedside stand_____ Closet _____

Drawers_____ Bathroom _____ Mealtime_____ Visiting hours _____

Information obtained from: Patient_____ Spouse _____ Parent: M_____ F_____ Other _____

Other observations and comments: _____

_____

Show all body marks: scars, bruises, cuts, decubiti, ulcers, and discolorations (birth marks should not be shown).

Signed _____

Figure 32-3 An admission checklist.

Drawing Conclusions

1. What types of activities that occur in a hospital might require explanation to a client who has never before been in a hospital?

    _____

    _____

    _____

2. Why is it important to note all scars, bruises, decubiti, ulcers, and other body marks on admission?

    _____

    _____

    _____

Critical Thinking

Personnel Issues

Place yourself in the role of a manager in a health care facility. It is time for the first 3-month employee review in the following two situations. Prepare a written evaluation of at least two paragraphs for each of the two individuals described. You may create additional facts as desired for your evaluation. These situations may also be used for role play.

Situation One

Overall, the performance of Nancy BeGood is adequate for this level of job entry. However, there are some problems that have been noted by you and mentioned by her fellow workers. These problems include that Nancy is late for work one to two times weekly, always by just a few minutes. Additionally, she takes a few extra minutes for break several times each week, again usually less than 5 minutes. She does not show initiative in finding tasks to be performed when she finishes the assigned work. She uses slang terms instead of correct medical terminology when talking with staff members, doctors, and patients.

Examining the Evidence

1. Which issue about Nancy's behavior do you consider the most important to correct? Explain why.

    _____

    _____

    _____

2. Why is arriving late to work or returning late from break a problem even when it is only a few minutes?

    _____

    _____

    _____

3. What would be an appropriate method and time period in which to follow-up on this employee review?

_____

_____

_____

Situation Two

John Longface is having some personal problems at home. His work has been above average in the past but is now being performed inadequately. This problem started about 2 weeks before this review. His performance is too poor for you to allow it to continue. The most recent incident was his absence from work without notifying anyone that he would be gone. When you called his residence to see if he had left for work, you were informed by his wife that he was in bed and did not plan to come in.

Examining the Evidence

1. Explain why it is unacceptable to let personal problems affect work performance.

_____

_____

_____

2. How do people "rise above" or "put aside" personal problems when at work?

_____

_____

_____

3. What would be an appropriate method and time in which to follow up on this employee review?

_____

_____

_____

33 Environmental Careers

Vapid Vocabulary

Before reading the chapter, review the glossary terms from the chapter in the word search puzzle below. Define each of the terms in the space provided.

```
U  N  I  V  E  R  S  E  Y  R  I  O  V  R  E  S  E  R  S  T
U  T  T  E  O  R  L  R  O  U  I  T  L  T  N  U  R  C  I  I
Q  I  R  I  R  E  A  E  T  I  E  I  L  E  T  V  N  R  P  O
S  I  N  T  R  L  C  R  I  C  N  N  N  T  N  O  R  I  T  I
T  U  O  N  L  Q  E  T  U  A  I  I  U  E  I  I  N  T  E  U
I  N  T  I  I  U  N  L  T  N  P  R  T  T  E  N  I  M  N  T
U  E  C  T  T  R  I  T  C  O  T  I  I  I  R  I  I  I  I  H
S  N  O  I  S  A  I  I  P  S  E  R  U  T  I  I  A  U  T  R
A  I  N  T  N  S  N  U  U  R  T  V  Q  I  T  N  N  T  N  P
E  I  A  U  A  E  L  M  I  U  N  I  L  V  V  S  N  E  A  S
I  T  P  U  R  A  T  I  N  O  A  U  T  S  T  U  T  I  R  E
L  T  L  A  T  S  M  Y  R  R  N  L  T  I  T  T  T  I  A  T
N  T  T  I  O  U  M  R  P  I  R  I  T  C  I  N  A  O  U  I
E  E  O  T  N  I  U  N  I  T  T  T  U  A  R  I  U  T  Q  T
A  N  N  N  P  Q  N  I  E  L  U  S  A  H  T  T  T  P  N  Y
R  E  H  A  B  I  L  I  T  A  T  I  O  N  I  T  T  I  I  E
L  O  S  O  R  E  A  T  T  N  R  I  T  A  O  A  T  R  T  U
A  I  M  N  R  L  A  M  I  T  P  O  O  C  I  T  O  U  E  A
O  U  R  T  V  O  M  U  Q  S  R  E  T  I  T  L  Q  O  N  I
Q  A  R  T  N  I  S  I  I  N  E  A  T  U  I  E  N  L  O  R
```

1. Aerosol- _____

2. Ancillary- _____

3. Incinerate- _____

4. Nutrition- _____

5. Optimal- _____

6. Population- _____

7. Quarantine- _____

8. Rehabilitation- _____

9. Reservoir- _____

10. Universe- _____

Key Search

Find the Key Terms of the chapter by matching the terms to the definitions in the space provided.

Term Tank	
Biosphere	Mutagen
Decibel	Particulate
Ecosystem	Pesticide
Hydrocarbon	Pollution

DEFINITION	KEY TERM
Composed of separate particles or pieces	
Living organisms and nonliving elements interacting in a specific area	
Condition of being defiled or impure	
Poison used to destroy pests of any kind	
Part of the universe, including the air, earth, and water, in which living organisms exist	
Physical or chemical agent that induces genetic mutation or change	
Organic compound made of hydrogen and carbon only	
Unit used to express ratio of power between two sounds	

Just the Facts

1. Most _ _ _ _ _ _ _ _ _ workers are not seen by the person receiving the service.

2. _ _ Ⓞ _ _ _ _ _ _ _ supervise food operations to meet the patients' needs and provide counseling on nutrition.

3. The type of _ _ Ⓞ _ _ _ _ _ is determined by the physician's order and special needs of the patient.

4. The _ Ⓞ _ _ _ _ _ _ _ _ _ _ _ _ Ⓞ _ _ engineer analyzes contamination problems to establish methods and equipment to prevent pollution.

5. _ _ _ _ _ _ _ _ Ⓞ _ _ _ _ _ _ _ identify existing and potential hazards in conditions and practices.

6. _ _ _ _ _ _ Ⓞ _ _ _ _ analyze and regulate the quality of the environment as it is affected by living organisms.

7. _ _ _ _ _ _ _ _ _ _ services include groundskeeping, housekeeping, and other personnel needed to run a large institution.

8. The Ⓞ _ _ _ _ _ _ _ _ _ _ _ Ⓞ _ _ _ _ _ _ or operating room technologist maintains the sterile field during surgery and passes instruments to the surgeon.

9. _ _ _ _ _ _ _ Ⓞ Ⓞ _ _ _ _ _ _ _, or sterile supply technicians, sterilize, assemble, clean, and store diagnostic and surgical equipment.

10. The _ Ⓞ _ _ _ _ _ _ _ is the air, crust of the earth, and water.

Use the circled letters to form the answer to this jumble. Clue: What do more than 23 million Americans have in common?

_ _ _ _ _ _ _ _   _ _ _ _ _

Concept Applications

Identifying the Parts and Functions of the Chain of Life

Use Figure 33-6 in the textbook to label the diagram of the chain of life in Figure 33-1. In the spaces provided in Table 33-1, explain the role played by each of the parts of the chain in the recycling of the biosphere's resources.

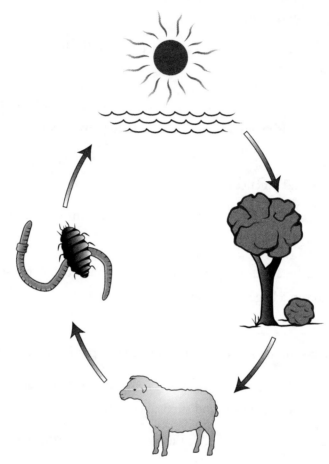

Figure 33-1

TABLE 33-1

Part of the Chain	Role in the Biosphere
1. Sunlight, water, air, organic compounds, and nutrients–	
2. Plants on land and water–	
3. Herbivores and carnivores–	
4. Decomposers–	

Using the Epidemiologic Approach

Use the epidemiologic approach provided in the textbook to identify and solve the health problem described.

Problem Description

Your club participated in the school picnic. To raise funds, you sold soft drinks. Other clubs provided hamburgers, pizza, several types of salad, cookies, and ice cream.

Approximately 2 hours after the picnic, 40 students became very ill and had to be taken to a local health care facility.

The administration decided that no more food-related activities would be allowed on the school campus. Your club would like the administration to reconsider.

You plan to investigate this problem. You may invent information resulting from your investigation needed to solve the problem. Complete the chart to show the solution you found following your imaginary investigation.

Epidemiologic Method	
Step one:	Identify the problem.
Step two:	Identify the illness.
Step three:	Identify the source of the problem.
Step four:	Prevent further incidence.

Applying Your Knowledge

1. What are three food-related sources of intestinal disorders?

   _____

   _____

   _____

2. How could the epidemiologic approach be used to trace the source of a breakout of hepatitis A to a restaurant worker who carries the virus?

   _____

   _____

   _____

3. For what other health-related problems could the epidemiologic approach be used?

   _____

   _____

   _____

Designing a Health Care Environment

Use the information you have learned from the chapter to design a health care environment that includes therapeutic and functional aspects such as color, decor, and furnishings. It should also provide organizational spaces to prevent clutter and promote safety considerations. You may design either a hospital room, a hospital unit (floor), a surgical or examination suite, or a facility of your choice. Your teacher may ask you to provide your design as a written description, poster, or three-dimensional model.

Environmental Careers

Environmental Skills and Qualities

List three personal qualities and skills that are important in environmental careers.

1. _____

2. _____

3. _____

Identifying Environmental Careers

Use the textbook to complete the missing information about environmental careers in Table 33-2.

TABLE 33-2

Career Title	Years of Education	Description of Job Duties and Opportunities	Credentials Required
		Modify facilities for environmental protection; recommend equipment to meet government standards	
		Analyze and regulate the quality of the environment; pollution analysis	
			MS or PhD preferred; registration available
		Counsel patients in methods to reduce weight	
		Provide equipment and supplies in facilities	

Applying Your Knowledge

1. Health care workers who provide services that are not generally seen by the public are called

   _____.

2. A 2-year associate degree is needed for the health care worker who plans menus and supervises the production of food and is called a _____.

3. Analysis of contamination problems and establishment of methods of their production is performed by the _____.

4. Health physics technicians are also called _____.

5. Certification as a specialist in public health may be granted for health care workers called

   _____.

Investigations

Water Analysis

Read all of the directions before beginning this activity. Laboratory activities should be completed only under the supervision of a qualified professional.

Equipment and Supplies

incubator
inoculating loop
litmus paper
microscope
Secchi disk
sterile agar plate
thermometer
water samples collected in sterile containers

Directions

1. Collect a water sample in a sterile container. Elements of the water that may indicate pollution include the presence of animal and plant life. The specimen must be collected in a sterile container to prevent contamination from other sources.

2. Observe and record the temperature of the water. Water temperature varies with the climate, oxygen content, and depth of the water sample.

3. Observe and record the turbidity of the water. The turbidity, or clarity, of the water can be determined by the amount of light that passes through it or by use of a Secchi disk. Water with high turbidity may be unacceptable for use by humans.

4. Observe and record the odor of the water. Odor may result from chemicals, organisms, or organic materials in the water. Odor does not necessarily indicate pollution of the water, but it is undesirable.

5. Using a microscope, observe the water and record the presence of life forms in the sample. The animals and plants that live in a body of water are indicators of its oxygen and other contents. Microscopic life forms may indicate that the water is unacceptable for use by humans.

6. Observe and record the uses of the water sample area. Water may be used for recreational or industrial purposes. Litter in the water may indicate pollution from inappropriate use.

7. Measure and record the pH of the water sample. Litmus paper can be used to indicate the concentration of acid or alkaline materials in the water sample. The acidity of the water determines whether algae will grow and the relative quantity of minerals or hardness of the water.

8. Prepare and incubate a streak culture plate to determine the presence of microscopic bacteria in the sample. Record results in Table 33-3.

9. Determine the acceptability of the water sample for its intended use. Drinking water should have a neutral pH, be free of microorganisms, have no odor, and be at an appropriate temperature.

Table 33-3   Water Analysis Comparison

Type of Water Sample	Tap	Pond
Date and site of water collection		
Temperature of water at time of collection		
Turbidity		
Odor		
Description of microscopic organisms		
Uses of the water sampled		
pH of water sample		
Description of streak plate growth		

Drawing Conclusions

1. Why is the presence of microscopic organisms in water important in determining whether it may be used for drinking and swimming?

   _____

   _____

   _____

2. Explain whether the water samples you tested are safe for drinking.

   _____

   _____

   _____

3. Which health professional collects and analyzes air and water samples under the supervision of the sanitarian?

   _____

   _____

   _____

4. What are three sources of water contamination?

   _____

   _____

   _____

Critical Thinking

Respiratory Effects of Chemical Exposure

The functional units of the respiratory system are directly exposed to the environment. The surface of the lungs provides the largest exposed area of the body. The surface area of the lungs is 70 to 100 m^2 compared with the surface area of the digestive system, which is $10m^2$, and the skin, which is only 2 m^2. Harmful exposure to poisonous substances occurs very quickly through the lung tissue.

Toxins or poisonous substances that can be inhaled are divided into the following categories:

1. Asphyxiates—gases that deprive the body of oxygen, such as carbon dioxide, nitrogen, cyanide, neon, and argon

2. Irritants—chemicals that irritate the air passages, such as chlorine, hydrochloric acid, and ammonia

3. Necrosis producers—gases that result in cell death, such as ozone and nitrogen dioxide

4. Fibrosis producers—substances that result in formation of fibrotic tissues, such as asbestos and silicates

5. Allergens—substances that produce an allergic response, such as isocyanates and sulfur dioxide

6. Carcinogens—substances that cause cancerous cells to form, such as cigarette smoke, asbestos, and arsenic

Examining the Evidence

1. Which of the toxin categories include most of the particulates in air pollution?

   _____

   _____

   _____

2. To which of the toxins listed are you exposed?

   _____

   _____

   _____

3. What are two methods you might use to limit your exposure to the toxins described?

   _____

   _____

   _____

4. Carbon monoxide is known to bind to the hemoglobin molecule 200 times more readily than oxygen. What effect does this have in the body?

   _____

   _____

   _____

5. What are two common sources of carbon monoxide?

   _____

   _____

   _____

Pneumonic Plague

Widespread panic broke out in one city in western India in September 1994 when an outbreak of pneumonic plague occurred. More than 200,000 people fled one city trying to avoid a national epidemic. By October, the World Health Organization announced that the plague was under control following the reported deaths of up to 300 people.

Pneumonic plague is caused by the bacteria *Yersinia pestis*. It affects animals such as rodents but can be transmitted to people by fleas. The infection can then be spread from one person to another by air droplets.

Examining the Evidence

1. The Centers for Disease Control and Prevention usually impose a quarantine to prevent the spread of an unknown or infectious agent. Why would this be an important method of treatment?

   _____

   _____

   _____

2. How might this plague be contained?

   _____

   _____

   _____

Radiation Testing

In October 1994, the President's Advisory Committee on Human Radiation Experiments revealed thousands of secret experiments using radiation that had been conducted between 1944 and 1974. Tests included the releasing of radioactive particles into the environment and the injection into human beings. Approximately 23,000 people were involved in these studies, some without their knowledge. The Departments of Energy and Defense still refuse to release all documents involved in the testing.

Examining the Evidence

1. Most individuals involved in secret tests would not know their risk of complications. Why do or do you not think that these individuals should be informed now?

   _____

   _____

   _____

2. One action under consideration by the committee is financial compensation of victims of testing. Why do or do you not agree with this action?

   _____

   _____

   _____

3. What kinds of safeguards protect the public from secret testing today?

_____

_____

_____

4. Research to discover at least one other type of environmental or public health risk caused by the action of the government or some other agency.

_____

_____

_____

34 Biotechnology Careers

Vapid Vocabulary

Before reading the chapter, review the glossary terms from the chapter in the word search puzzle below. Define each of the terms in the space provided.

```
D C E A E R L N E C N T R D E O X C I O
N T T L Y Y Y N I U E D S M S O E N E E
O I C A Y C G N C T I Y A Y I I N A T S
E T I A B I E L Y N A T R A L A N E R T
E A A E E G E E L A E I E C C A N A C Y
T I E E S I Y L N N T N T E E I T E L I
T E I N C N E E O I T A A R S R S A T E
N O A A L I E E C B E E O P A A C E C S
N R C N O C C Y P M P N E T D A O T O C
T I E O P I I E O O I O R I R O I D O I
D E A Y E L T P C C P E X T C E I A I X
T C A A S T G I D E I O O Y E O S I T C
A T C T A I E A E R R E N E E B B A L G
A A E T C A R T X E L A M I N A R O L E
N E A E P T E Y E A A E I I C I N E R E
A T C A O T I N T N N T I D E E I E Y D
C T E A E C O T P P E T Y E A N P E E R
R E O C O I E L I C S A C I E M A A N T
E E N B I O E O O N E E T O E A I Y T E
I N I E P A E N C C O A O T L E E T C R
```

1. Catalyst-_____

2. Clone- _____

3. Extract- _____

4. Laminar- _____

5. Laser- _____

6. Nucleic acid- _____

7. Oxidase- _____

8. Pipette- _____

9. Recombinant- _____

10. Transgenic- _____

Key Search

Find the Key Terms of the chapter by matching the terms to the definitions in the space provided.

Term Tank		
Artificial insemination	Eugenics	Selective breeding
Deoxyribonucleic acid	Fermentation	
Electrophoresis	Forensics	
Enzyme	Monoclonal antibody	

DEFINITION	KEY TERM
Protein that acts as a catalyst in the cell	
Choosing the parents of offspring to enhance development of desired traits	
Injection of semen into the uterine canal, unrelated to sexual intercourse	
Identical cells or cells originating from the same cell	
Large nucleic acid molecule that makes up chromosomes	
Chemical change that is brought about by the action of an enzyme or microorganism	
Pertaining to the courts of law	
Study of the methods for controlling the characteristics of humans	
Movement of charged suspended particles through a medium in responses to an electric field	

Just the Facts

1. Biotechnology applies scientific and engineering techniques to the manipulation of the
   _ _ _ Ⓞ _ of living organisms.

2. Scientists have been using natural techniques of biotechnology such as
   _ _ _ _ _ _ Ⓞ _ _ _ _ _, _ _ _ _ _ _ _ _ _ _ breeding,
   and _ _ _ _ _ _ Ⓞ _ _ _ insemination for many years.

3. _ _ _ Ⓞ _ _ guidelines for the transfer and manipulation of DNA have been established by the National Institutes of Health.

4. Biotechnologists may work in many fields of practice including research,
   _ Ⓞ _ _ _ _ _ _ _ _, _ _ _ _ _ _ _ _ _ _ _ _, and teaching.

5. Medical biotechnologists work with the production of _ _ _ _ _ _ _ _ _ Ⓞ
   for diagnosis or treatment of disease.

6. _ _ _ _ _ Ⓞ _ _ _ _ _ study patterns of inheritance and develop methods to influence genetic information.

7. _ _ _ _ _ _ _ _ _ _ _ Ⓞ _ _ _ _ _ _ _ is a molecule
   that, by the sequencing of its components, determines all of the characteristics of living things.

8. The Ⓞ _ _ _ _ _ _ _ _ _ _ _ _ Ⓞ _ _ _ _ _ is an international effort to identify and sequence all of the human chromosomes.

9. Some genetically modified foods in development include edible _ _ _ _ _ _ _ Ⓞ,
   therapeutic Ⓞ _ _ _ _ _ _ _, and _ _ _ _ _ _ _ _ Ⓞ _ produced by plants.

10. Some of the techniques of biotechnology include gene _ _ Ⓞ _ _ _ _ and gene
    _ _ _ _ _ _ _ _ or Ⓞ _ _ _ _ _ _ _ _ _ _ DNA.

Use the circled letters to form the answer to this jumble. Clue: What is the name of the biotechnology technique that may be used to identify suspects in a crime or determine paternity?

_ _ _ _ _ _ _ _ _ _ _ _ _ _ _ _

Concept Applications

Identifying the Structure of DNA

Use Figure 34-1 in the textbook to label the diagram of DNA in Figure 34-1.

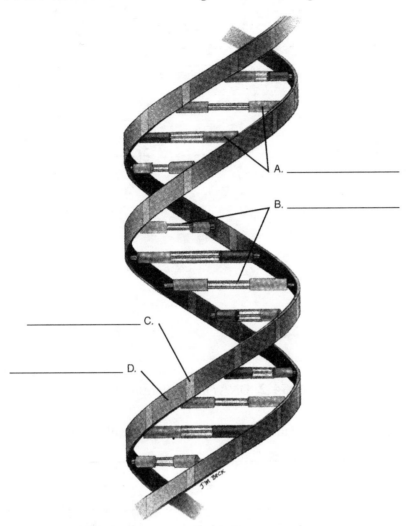

A. _____

B. _____

_____ C.

_____ D.

Figure 34-1 Courtesy of Joan M. Beck

Settling a Paternity Suit

Figure 34-2 is the DNA analysis results from a disputed paternity suit. The mother claims that one of the three men tested is the father of her child. Testing for blood type was inconclusive. The mother has blood type O. The child is blood type O. The three men have blood types A, B, and O.

Applying Your Knowledge

1. Why would the tests for blood type be inconclusive?

_____

_____

_____

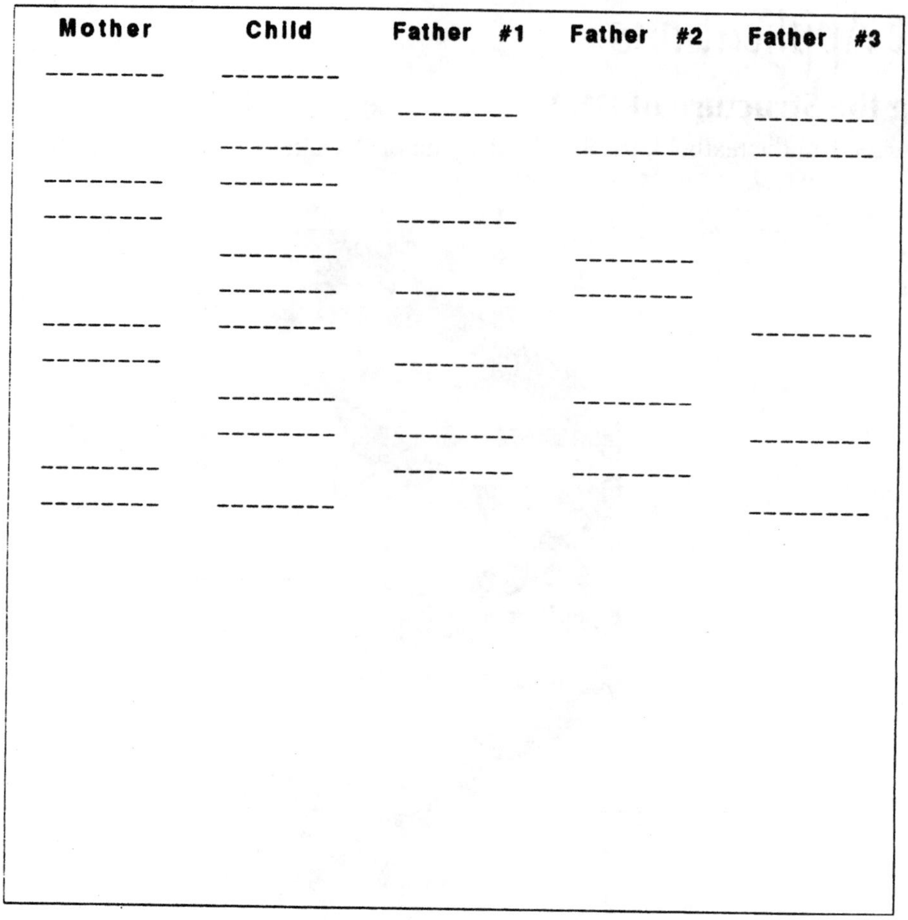

Figure 34-2 DNA *Electrophoresis Digest*

2. Which individual(s) may be eliminated as the potential father of the child?

_____

_____

_____

3. Which individual(s) may not be eliminated as the father of the child?

_____

_____

_____

Biotechnology Careers

Biotechnology Skills and Qualities

List three personal qualities and skills that are important in biotechnology careers.

1. _____

2. _____

3. _____

Identifying Biotechnology Careers

Use the textbook to complete the missing information about biotechnology careers in Table 34-1.

TABLE 34–1

Career Title	Years of Education	Description of Job Duties and Opportunities	Credentials Required
		Bioinstrumentation, biothermodynamics, biotransport, biomechanics	
		Conduct research in cell genetics; may work in research, medicine, or forensics	
	Apprenticeship		

Applying Your Knowledge

1. Health care workers who design new devices such as robotic surgical instruments are called

   _____.

2. Information regarding the genetic makeup of an individual may be determined by the

   _____.

3. A 4-year degree in biotechnology qualifies an individual for work as a(n)

   _____.

Investigations

Performing a DNA Extraction

Read all of the directions before beginning this activity. Laboratory activities should be completed only under the supervision of a qualified professional.

IEquipment and Supplies

alcohol
250-mL beaker
dishwashing liquid
eyedropper
glass rod
hot water bath
nonpathogenic bacteria (yeast may be used)
nutrient broth (water for yeast)
test tube
test tube holder
thermometer

Directions

1. Maintain medical asepsis by practicing good handwashing technique.
2. Prepare a broth of nonpathogenic bacteria or mix yeast in water at 50°–60° C.
3. Pour approximately 10 mL of bacterial broth into a clean test tube.
4. Add approximately 5 mL of dishwashing liquid into the test tube.
5. Place the test tube into a hot water bath for 15 minutes. Do not exceed 60° C.
6. Use an eyedropper to add alcohol to cover the top of the solution.
7. Gently stir a glass rod into the solution, through the alcohol.
8. Continue to stir the glass rod through the alcohol into the solution.
9. Record your observations.
10. Clean materials as directed by your instructor and place in the designated location.

Drawing Conclusions

1. What are the fibers that collect around the glass tube?

   _____

   _____

   _____

2. Why must the glass rod be turned gently in the solution?

   _____

   _____

   _____

3. What is the purpose of each of the reagents used in the extraction?

   _____

   _____

   _____

Critical Thinking

Genetic Testing

Many genetic tests can now be performed using a simple blood test. Some examples include:

- detection of the Tay-Sachs gene in a carrier (see Chapter 15 for more information regarding Tay-Sachs)
- determination of nonpaternity of an alleged father with 99% accuracy
- detection of Down syndrome and neural tube defects in a fetus by testing the mother's blood (see Chapter 18 for more information regarding Down syndrome and neural tube defects)

Examining the Evidence

1. Why does a paternity test exclude an alleged father but not identify one directly?

   _____

   _____

   _____

2. What are three advantages of knowing that a fetus has a disorder such as a neural tube defect or Down syndrome?

   _____

   _____

   _____

3. Why do some people not want to have genetic testing done to determine any defects that might be present in a fetus?

   _____

   _____

   _____

Cloning Controversy

Scientists at George Washington University cloned a human embryo in 1993. In this case, flawed embryos were divided and allowed to grow to the 32-cell stage. Embryos that contain 32 cells are often used for in vitro implantation. These cells were discarded after 6 days. No clear guidelines exist for this type of research and human experimentation. The American Fertility Society (AFS) has set voluntary guidelines that prohibit human embryos from being developed in a test tube more than 14 days.

Examining the Evidence

1. What might be some of the concerns regarding the cloning of human embryos?

   _____

   _____

   _____

2. What guidelines could be established to maintain an ethical policy regarding the cloning of human embryos?

_____

_____

_____

3. How can the public's perception of biotechnology research be improved?

_____

_____

_____

Exercises in Genetic Counseling

Consider the following situations that might occur in a genetic counseling center. Describe what action you feel would be appropriate for the counselor to follow.

Situation One

The patient comes in for testing to determine whether her fetus inherited two genes for cystic fibrosis. Testing is done on the woman and her husband. The blood tests show that the fetus does have the condition but that the husband is not a carrier. The woman forbids the counselor from telling the husband that the child is not his.

How would you respond if you were the genetic counselor?

_____

_____

_____

Situation Two

The patients have a genetic condition of polydactyly. They want their fetus tested for the condition. They inform the counselor of their intention to abort any fetus that is "normal," or without the condition. They feel that they do not want to raise a child who is different from them.

How would you respond if you were the genetic counselor?

_____

_____

_____

Situation Three

The patient carries the genetic trait for sickle cell anemia. She tells you that she will abort any fetus that carries the gene because she wants the condition to end with her generation.

How would you respond if you were the genetic counselor?

_____

_____

_____